Low carb cookbook

To start losing weight

James L. Gay

Contents

1. INTRODUCTION   1

2. HIGH PROTEIN, LOW CARB FOODS   83

3. WHAT YOU CAN AND CAN'T EAT   86

4. RISKS OF HIGH PROTEIN, LOW CARB DIETS   89

5. A WHOLICIOUS APPROACH TO HEALTHY   92
EATING

Chapter One

INTRODUCTION

High protein, low carb diets can work for weight loss in the short -term, yet they do have risks so it is important to weigh up the proof before you decide if it's a good option for you.

While weight gain as a rule happens over numerous years ,many of us want a convenient solution solution to trim down. This may be one of the reasons that high protein, low carb diets have become well known again they can give fast results in the short-term. But is losing a few kilograms in the shortterm worth damagingyour healthin the long-term?

If you call it the Atkins Diet, South Beach Diet, Dukan Diet or Paleo they are largely very much the same. They tend to emphasise:

A high intake of animal proteins like red meat, chicken, fish and eggs; Combined with a sharp decrease in sugars including breads, rice, pastas, grains, legumes and organic products; and

In a few cases, a high admission of fat is likewise encouraged, especially from nuts, seeds, extra virgin cold pressed olive oil, coconut oils, full-cream dairy products, butter and ghee.

While high protein diets might be getting some things right by encouraging bounty of vegetables and advocating no refined foods; there are other parts that you may need to reconsider.

How High Protein, Low Carb Diets Works

They cut out the bad carbs . One of the fundamental reasons these diets work in the short term is that they stay away from all high-energy, low-nutrient refined carbs like soft drinks, cakes, lollies, biscuits, hot chips and crisps. But thisadvice is not unique to highprotein, low carb diets it is a good idea for anyone wanting to lose weight and live a healthy lifestyle to reduce their intake of refined carbohydrates.

They cut out entire food groups. By cutting out any food gatherings (like wholegrains, legumes and dairy) you restrict your food choices and therefore eat less. This may seem favorable, notwithstanding, it can result in you missing out on important food nutrients!

They dampen your appetite . Proteins and fats tend to be more filling, as they can take more time to digest.

Nonetheless, don't forget that wholegrain carbohydrates and vegetables are very filling too because they're packed with fiber, hosing yourappetite so you do not crave as much food.

The main worry with high protein, low carb counts calories is that they are difficult to keep up with over the long term and they tend to be nutritionally unbalanced.

Hard to maintain . Cutting out carbs does mean you are likely to eat less energy generally speaking. But this is almostimpossible to maintain over the long term. A study tracking 3000 individuals who lost over 30kg and kept it off for more than 5 years, found that less than 1 percent had followed a high protein, low carb diet. The rest reported reliably eating a low fat, high carbohydrate diet combined with regular work out. The high protein calorie counters also kept up with their weight misfortune for less time than the others and were likewise less physically

dynamic, possible due to having lower energy levels.

Out of whack and lopsided . While there is no standard definition for 'high protein' some of the well known weight control plans can have protein levels more than twofold the sum exhorted in the Australian Dietary Guidelines. They also tend to have very high levels of soaked fat and dietary cholesterol and cut out or limit whole grains, dull vegetables and fruits, which are all significant weapons against way of life disease, including heart sickness, stroke and diabetes.

This lopsided approach to eating can have aftereffects and more serious long-term health impacts.

1,400-CALORIE HIGH- PROTEIN LOW- CARB MEAL PLAN

Jumpstart weight misfortune with this 1,400-calorie high-protein, low-carb meal plan.

A low -carb diet joined with a low-calorie diet can be one of the most effective ways to lose weight quickly, agreeing to research. Better yet, a lowcarb, low-calorie diet that's also high in protein can make weight loss even easier. Protein does a great work of helping you feel more full for longer, which is particularly accommodating when cutting calories and restricting your carb intake, which in turn decreases how much fiber you're getting. While low-carb diets like the ketogenic diet and Atkins diet restrict carbs to as low as 20 grams for each day, you don't have to go that low to see weight reduction benefits. Eating too few sugars can actually make weight misfortune harder because you miss out on key supplements, like fiber from whole grains and legumes, that help you to feel full and fulfilled on less calories. So what can you actually eat on a high-protein, low-carb diet? Thankfully, there are a lot of delicious, healthy foods to fill your day with while following this eating plan.

In this high -protein, lowcarb weekly meal plan, we keep the carbs at no more than 120 grams per day while still meeting the recommended amount of fiber every day (30 grams) from fiber- rich products of the soil, like berries, edamame and hearty kale. You'll still see some traditional carbs in the arrangement, like beans and chickpeas, because they are healthy foods that you don't have to completely reject in order to eat low-carb. To make up for the lower amount of carbs, we packed in high-protein foods (like chicken, eggs and lean beef) to exceed the daily recommended amount of 50 grams per day, and added healthy fat sources (like almonds, olive oil and peanut butter) to get the calories up to 1,400. Bundled into an easy-to-follow dinner plan, with simple feast prep tips you can follow at the starting of the week to set yourself up for success during the occupied weekdays, this low-calorie, low-carb, highprotein combination will help you get in shape without feeling deprived or starved. With the calorie count set at 1,400 calories, you can expect to lose a sound 1 to 2 pounds per week. Looking for a lower calorie level? See this supper planat 1,200 calories.

How to Meal-Prep Your Week of Meals:

1. Make the Flourless Banana Chocolate Chip Mini Muffins to have for breakfast on Days 2 and 3 and as a nibble on Days 1 and 4.

2. Prepthe Chicken Satay Bowls with Spicy Peanut Sauce to have for lunch on Days 2, 3, 4 and 5.

Day 1

In request to keep your carbs on the lower end , you are most frequently cutting out fiber-rich food varieties like whole grains, beans and legumes. Therefore, we made sure to pack this lowcarb plan with at least 30 grams of fiber per day, mostly from fruits, vegetables and some entire grains and legumes. This ensures that you are still getting the nutritional benefits of fiber

(stomach health and fulfillment) while keeping carbs in check.

Breakfast (355 calories, 16 g protein, 32 g carbs)

• 1 serving"Egg in a Hole" Peppers with Avocado Salsa

• 2 clementines

A.M. Sn ack (238calories, 7 g protein, 27 g carbs)

1 cup blueberries

20 unsalted almonds

Lunch (322calories, 22 g protein, 11 g carbs)

• 1 serving Salmon Salad-Stuffed Avocado P.M. Snack (78 calories, 1 g protein, 11 g carbs)

• 1 Flourless Banana Chocolate Chip Mini Muffin

Dinner (389 calories, 10 g protein, 36 g carbs) 1 servingWhiteBean Sage Cauliflower Gnocchi 2 cups mixed salad greens

1 Tbsp.Caesar Salad Dressing

¼ cup chopped tomato

¼ cup chopped cucumber 3 Tbsp. diced avocado

Toss salad greens with dressing, tomato, cucumber and avocado.

Daily Totals: 1,382 calories, 69 g fat, 32 g fiber, 103 g carbohydrates, 50 g protein, 1,565 mg sodium Day 2

To keep carbs low today , we included these sound flourless banana chocolate chip muffins made from oats, banana and eggs, and traded in zucchini noodles for regular pasta in tonight's supper. To make sure you are still getting adequate amounts of both carbohydrates and fiber, we filled in the rest of the day with nutrient-rich food sources like blackberries, edamame and a serving of entire wheat baguette at supper to sop up any of the scrumptious leftover juice from the scampi.

Br eakfast (352 calories, 27 g protein, 45 g carbs)

2Flourless Banana Chocolate Chip Mini Muffins 1 cup raspberries

1 cup nonfat Greek yogurt

A.M. Snack (62calories, 2 g protein, 14 g carbs)

• 1 cup blackberries Lunch (351 calories, 28 g protein, 14 g carbs)

• 1 serving Chicken Satay Bowls with Spicy Peanut Sauce P.M. Snack (200calories, 16 gprotein, 18 g carbs)

• 1 cup shelled edamame, prepared with coarse salt and pepper, to taste

D inner (448 calories, 31 gprotein, 34 g carbs)

1 serving

Shrimp Scampi Zoodles 1 serving

Shrimp Scampi Zoodles

inch) cut whole-wheat baguette

1 tsp. olive oil to brush on baguette

Daily Totals: 1,414 calories, 105 g protein, 125 g carbs, 33 g fiber, 56 g fat, 1,811 mg sodium

Day 3

Just a single cup of raspberries contains 8 grams of filling fiber with just 15 grams of carbs, which is why you'll see them often on this simple high- protein, lowcarb meal plan. High-fiber food varieties tend to be more filling than low-fiber foods, so you're likely to eat less and stay fulfilled longer, which is especially important when cutting calories to lose weight.

Breakfast (352 calories, 27 g protein, 45 g carbs)

2Flourless Banana Chocolate Chip Mini Muffins 1 cup raspberries

1 cup non-fat Greek yogurt

A.M. Sn ack (262calories, 8 g protein, 25 g carbs) 25 unsalted almonds

2 clementines Lunch (351calories, 28 g protein, 14 gcarbs) • 1 serving Chicken Satay Bowls with Spicy Peanut Sauce

P.M. Sn ack (62 calories, 2 g protein, 14 g carbs)

• 1 cup blackberries Dinner (378calories, 32 gprotein, 31 g carbs)

• 1 serving Pork Paprikash with Cauliflower "Rice" • 1 serving Roasted Fresh Green Beans

Daily Totals: 1,406 calories, 97 g protein, 128 g carbs, 43 g fiber, 62 g fat, 1,307 mg sodium Day 4

Moreover to being an incredible source of protein , which helps keep up with muscle mass while you're losing weight, salmon is a great source of omega-3 fatty acids, a fundamental fatty corrosive that you must get in your diet. Early research additionally shows that salmon eaters had lower fasting insulin levels, which can help keep your blood sugar in check and reduce your hazard for diabetes. Roasted salmon is served over low-carb veggie-licious kale and chickpeas-a healthy carb you can definitely still be eating, even when following a low-carb diet.

Br eakfast (269calories, 26 g protein, 33 g carbs)

1 cup nonfat plain Greek yogurt 1 cup raspberries

1 tsp. honey

1 Tbsp. chia seeds

A.M. Snack (262 calories, 18 gprotein, 32 g carbs) 1 cup shelled edamame, prepared with coarse salt and pepper, to taste 1 cup blackberries

Lunch (351calories, 28 g protein, 14 g carbs) • 1 serving Chicken Satay Bowls with Spicy Peanut Sauce

P.M. Snack (78calories, 1 g protein, 11 g carbs) • 1 Flourless Banana Chocolate Chip Mini Muffin

Dinner (447 calories, 37 g protein, 23 g carbs) • 1 serving Roasted Salmon with Smoky Chickpeas and Greens

Daily Totals: 1,407 calories, 111 g protein, 114 g carbs, 39 g fiber, 57 g fat, 1,505 mg sodium Day 5

Our high -protein weight-loss meal plan includes fiber-rich carbohydrates, similar to those from berries, white beans and broccoli. Supper tonight packs in 15 grams of protein, which helps you feel full as well as also may help with weight misfortune. In one study, researchers found that for every 10 grams of solvent fiber eaten over the course of a day, there was a corresponding 3.7 percent decrease in abdominal fat.

Breakfast (259calories, 15 g protein, 10 g carbs) • 1 serving Low-Carb Bacon and Broccoli Egg Burrito

A.M. Sn ack (218 calories, 7 g protein, 20 g carbs)

1 cup raspberries

20 unsalted almonds

Lunch (351calories, 28 g protein, 14 gcarbs)

• 1 servingChicken Satay Bowls with Spicy Peanut Sauce

P.M. Snack (129 calories, 6 g protein, 14 g carbs) 1/4 cup hummus 4 celery stalks, cut into stalks

Dinner (442calories, 15 g protein, 50 g carbs)

• 1 serving Vegan Pesto Spaghetti Squash with Mushrooms and Sun-Dried Tomatoes

• 2/3 cup no-salt-added canned white beans, rinsed

Stir beans into an individual portion of the spaghetti squash and sauce.

Daily Totals: 1,407 calories, 111 g protein, 114 g carbs, 39 g fiber, 57 g fat, 1,505 mg sodium Day 6

Yes , you can still eat cheese and lose weight! String cheese is an extraordinary noontime snack, particularly when matched with fiber-rich raspberries. The combination of protein and fiber increases satisfaction and can lessen appetite at your next meal.

Br eakfast (269 calories, 26 g protein, 33 g carbs)

1 cup nonfat plain Greek yogurt 1 cup raspberries

1 tsp. honey 1 Tbsp. chia seeds

A.M. Snack (128 calories, 6 g protein, 22 g carbs)

1 little apple

1 string cheese

Lunch (351 calories, 22 g protein, 14 gcarbs) • 1 serving Chicken Satay Bowls with Spicy Peanut Sauce

P.M. Sn ack (180calories, 6 g protein, 19 g carbs)

1 cup raspberries

15 unsalted almonds

Dinner (479calories, 25 gprotein, 28 g carbs)

• 1 serving Taco Lettuce Wraps

• 1 serving Pineapple and Avocado Salad

Meal -Prep Tip: Save 1 serving of the Taco Lettuce Wraps to have for lunch on Day 7. When preparing the Pineapple and Avocado Salad, set aside 1/4 of an avocado and 1/2 cup pineapple before dressing with the vinaigrette to have for lunch on Day 7.

Daily Totals: 1,406 calories, 91 g protein, 115 g carbs, 39 g fiber, 7o g fat, 1,170 mg sodium Day 7

Lettuce takes the place of tortillas in our low -carb, gluten-free taco lettuce wraps. Stuffed with lean ground hamburger, jicama, avocado and salsa and a whopping 23 grams protein per serving, this lunch will keep you feeling full for hours.

Br eakfast (278 calories, 19 g protein, 22 g carbs) • 1 serving Spring Green Frittata • 1 cup raspberries

A.M. Snack (154calories, 5 g protein, 5 g carbs) • 20 unsalted almonds

Lunch (431 calories, 25 g protein, 28 g carbs)

1 serving

Taco Lettuce Wraps 1/4 avocado, sliced 1/2 cup cut pineapple

Combine avocado and pineapple with 1 tsp. lime juice and a squeeze of salt. P.M. Snack (62 calories, 2 g protein, 14 gcarbs)

• 1 cup blackberries

D inner (480calories, 33 g protein, 45 g carbs) • 1 serving Zucchini Lasagna ••inch) slice whole-wheat baguette

Daily Totals: 1,405 calories, 84 g protein, 113 g carbs, 35 g fiber, 71 g fat, 1,685 mg sodium

HIGH PROTEIN LOWCARB DIET RECIPES 1. Edamame Spaghetti With Kale CilantroPesto This bean pasta boasts just

22 grams of carbs per serving and keeps you full longer than other white and wheat pastas.

Serves: 4

Start to Finish: 18 minutes Prep: 10 minutes

Cook: 8 minutes

Ingredients:

1 cup of kale, tightly packed

1 cup of cilantro, firmly packed

1/4 cup of slivered almonds, toasted 1 garlic clove

1 serrano chile

1 tablespoon lime juice Dash of salt

1/4 cup of parmesan, grated 1/2 cup of olive oil

1handle ginger, sliced into shards Olive oil

2carrots, sliced into ribbons

1/4 cup of shredded coconut, toasted 1box (8 oz) Explore Cuisine Edamame Spaghetti

Instructions:

1) Blend first seven ingredients in a food processor. Add cheese. Stream in olive oil. Sauté ginger in oil until crispy.

2) Boil 8 cups of water and pour in organic edamame spaghetti. Cook for 8 minutes. Drain. 3)Toss together edamame spaghetti with carrots and pesto. Top with ginger and toasted coconut. Nutrition Information (per serving): Calories: 471; Carbs: 29 g; Fat: 27 g; Protein: 29 g

2. Seared Peppercorn Ahi Tuna with ArugulaSalad This is an easy, light summer recipe that anybody can make and enjoy

at home.

Skill level: Intermediat e Serves: 2 people

Start to Finish: 17 mins Prep: 5 mins

Cook: 12 mins

Ingr edients:

2(5 ounce) ahi tuna steaks 1 teaspoon kosher salt 1/4 teaspoon cayenne pepper 2 tablespoons olive oil

1 tablespoon black peppercorn 1 teaspoon Zuzu sauce

Hannah An's Signature Garlic Lime Sauce

Instructions:\s1) Role the fish steaks in the salt, cayenne pepper, and dark peppercorn blend. Put olive oil in a skillet over medium-high heat.

2) Gently place the seasoned tuna in the skillet and cook to desired doneness. Cooking all sides evenly (1 1/2 minutes per side for rare). Slice tuna steaks in an upward direction in meager slices and top with Zuzu sauce.

3) Served with Fresh Arugula Salad and Tiato Leaf

Nutritional Information (per serving): Calories 302 ; Carbohydrate 2.9 g; Fat 9.2 g; Protein 51.3 g

3. Asparagus Wrapped in Chili Spiced Bacon

Asparagus wrapped in chili -spiced bacon is a simple dish that packs the flavor. It's a great snack option, consolidating vegetables and bacon to guarantee you're getting enough fat while skimping on the carbs.

Skill level: Beginner Serves: 4 servings

Start to Finish: 32 minutes Prep: 20 minutes Cook: 12 minutes

Ingredients:

1 teaspoon Chili Powder

1/2 teaspoon Sucralose Based Sweetener (Sugar Substitute) (Sugar Substitute) 4 slices bacon

24 spears Asparagus

Instructions:

1) Soak 16 wooden toothpicks in warm water for 20 minutes.

2) Preheat grill. Place a sheet of wax paper on a sheet container and set aside. Consolidate the bean stew powder and sugar substitute in a small bowl.

3) Cut bacon strips in half. Lay them on the sheet pan and dust with the chili powder mixture.

4) Wrap three asparagus lances together with one cut of bacon (with the dusted side facing towards the asparagus); securing each end with a toothpick. You ought to have 8 packets.

5) Grill uncovered over medium-low heat for 12 minutes turning halfway through or until bacon is crisp.

6) Discard toothpicks and serve immediately. Each serving is 2 wraps. Nutritional information

(per serving): Calories: 128; Net Carbs: 2.6 g; Fat: 10.2 g; Protein: 5g

4. Cauliflower Rice

This flavorful side dish will satisfy your "carb tooth" without any of the bloat. Skill level: Intermediate

Serves: 4-6

Start to Finish: 25 minutes Prep: 3 minutes

Cook: 22 minutes

Ingredients:

For Joes:

1 tablespoon olive oil

1 medium yellow onion, finely diced 2 garlic cloves, cleaved or minced

1 pound ground beef (or protein of decision: ground turkey, cooked lentils, or crumbled tempeh also work great) (or protein of decision: ground turkey, cooked lentils, or crumbled tempeh also work great)

1 to 2 teaspoons chile powder 2 teaspoons dried oregano

1 teaspoon sea salt 1/4 cup tomato paste 1/4 cup tomato paste\sounce) can tomato sauce

1 tablespoon Dijon mustard 1 cup water, optional

Garnishes: sliced toasted almonds, chopped fresh cilantro and/or parsley, optional

F or Rice:

1head cauliflower

2 tablespoons extravirgin olive oil 1 cup finely diced onion

2 cloves garlic, chopped or minced

Instructions:\s1) Start the rice by chopping the cauliflower florets and some of the stems into little pieces and pulse them in a food processor until they are the consistency of rice. Do not over-chop.

2) In a large skillet, heat 2 tablespoons of oil over low to medium heat and add the 1 cup onions and 2 cloves of garlic. Stir well and cook for 3 minutes.

3) Add the cauliflower rice from the food processor and cook for 10- 15minutes, till you feel it's fully cooked and flavors are well combined.

4) Meanwhile, heat the remaining tablespoon of oil in a separate container over medium-low heat.

5) Sauté the medium onion for around 10 minutes, until translucent. 6)Add the remaining garlic and sauté for 1 more minute.

7) Add protein of decision, chile powder, oregano, and salt and stir.

8) Add the tomato glue, tomato sauce, and mustard; mix and cook for 5 minutes.

9) Add water, up to a cup, as expected to make a sauce; mix and cook another 5 minutes, until protein is cooked through.

10) Serve promptly on top of cauliflower rice, and garnish as desired. Nutritional information (per serving): Calories: 321; Carbs: 13g; Fat: 23 g; Protein: 19 g

5. Spicy Turkey Lettuce Cups

This is a simple to -get ready, delicious and filling meal that has a low calorie count. If you like eating turkey burgers or tacos, these are the perfect low carb/low calorie substitute! They will fulfill your craving without sabotaging your weight loss.

1. Fish

Certain types of seafood are lauded as protein powerhouses , such as yellowfin tuna, halibut, and tilapia. Try Bahian Halibut, a well-seasoned Caribbean dish with coconut flavors; it offers 48.7g of protein, 18.6g of fat, 1.1g of fiber, 4.6g of net carbs, and 400 calories per serving. Bring Tuna-Celery Salad to lunch and enjoy a protein-filled noontime feast; one serving offers 37g of protein.

2. Tofu

Tofu is an excellent vegetarian protein to add to a dish as it easily absorbs whatever flavors it's cooked with. Flavor up heated tofu with a zesty kick such as a chipotle marinade or a Moroccan rub. For a savory Meatless Monday supper, try Tofu Pad Thai, which contains 20.5g of protein, 26.9g of fat, 6.9g of fiber, 14.1g of net carbs, and 374.6 calories.

3. Eggs

The poster child of protein , one egg offers 6g of complete protein. This means it gives all the amino acids humans need in their diet. Jump start your day with a protein-packed dish such as Eggs Scrambled with Cheddar, Swiss Chard and Canadian Bacon. This entrée includes 32.6g of protein, 36.9g of fat, 1.2g of fiber, 3.6g of net carbs, and 482.9 calories.

4. Nuts

Nuts are a high protein , low carb snack that offer heart-solid fats and a lot of protein. In particular, peanuts, cashews, and almonds are great wagers for high-protein snacks. The Atkins Chocolate Peanut Butter Pretzel Bar packs a whopping 16g of protein between nibbles of real roasted peanuts, pretzels, and smooth peanut butter. You can also snatch a small bunch of Atkins Sweet and Salty Trail Mix, which is equal parts salty and sweet, with 7g of protein.

5. Chicken

Chicken is a great high protei n food. For dinner, try Green Goddess Grilled Chicken, which packs in 53g of protein, 16.9g of fat, 1.4g of net carbs, and 382.4calories Chicken Salad makes for a filling lunch, thanks to over 50g of protein per serving. Use a lettuce wrap for an added crunch.

1,400-CALORIE HIGH- PROTEIN LOW- CARB MEAL PLAN

Jumpstart weight misfortune with this 1,400-calorie high-protein, low-carb meal plan.

A low -carb diet joined with a low-calorie diet can be one of the most effective ways to lose weight quickly, agreeing to research. Better yet, a lowcarb, low-calorie diet that's also high in protein can make weight loss even easier. Protein does a great work of helping you feel more full for longer, which is particularly accommodating when cutting calories and restricting your carb intake, which in turn decreases how much fiber you're getting. While low-carb diets like the ketogenic diet and Atkins diet restrict carbs to as low as 20 grams for each day, you don't have to go that low to see weight reduction benefits. Eating too few sugars can actually make weight misfortune harder because you miss out on key supplements, like fiber from whole grains and legumes, that help you to feel full and fulfilled on less calories. So what can you actually eat on a high-protein, low-carb diet? Thankfully, there are a lot of delicious, healthy foods to fill your day with while following this eating plan.

In this high -protein, lowcarb weekly meal plan, we keep the carbs at no more than 120 grams per day while still meeting the recommended amount of fiber every day (30 grams) from fiber- rich products of the soil, like berries, edamame and hearty kale. You'll still see some traditional carbs in the arrangement, like beans and chickpeas, because they are healthy foods that you don't have to completely reject in order to eat low-carb. To make up for the lower amount of carbs, we packed in high-protein foods (like chicken, eggs and lean beef) to exceed the daily recommended amount of 50 grams per day, and added healthy fat sources (like almonds, olive oil and peanut butter) to get the calories up to 1,400. Bundled into an easy-to-follow dinner plan, with simple feast prep tips you can follow at the starting of the week to set yourself up\sfor success during the occupied weekdays, this low-calorie, low-carb, highprotein combination will help you get in shape without feeling deprived or starved. With the calorie count set at

1,400 calories, you can expect to lose a sound 1 to 2 pounds per week. Looking for a lower calorie level? See this supper planat 1,200 calories.

How to Meal-Prep Your Week of Meals:

1. Make the Flourless Banana Chocolate Chip Mini Muffins to have for breakfast on Days 2 and 3 and as a nibble on Days 1 and 4.

2. Prepthe Chicken Satay Bowls with Spicy Peanut Sauce to have for lunch on Days 2, 3, 4 and 5.

Day 1

In request to keep your carbs on the lower end , you are most frequently cutting out fiber-rich food varieties like whole grains, beans and legumes. Therefore, we made sure to pack this lowcarb plan with at least 30 grams of fiber per day, mostly from fruits, vegetables and some entire grains and legumes. This ensures that you are still getting the nutritional benefits of fiber

(stomach health and fulfillment) while keeping carbs in check.

Breakfast (355 calories, 16 g protein, 32 g carbs) (355 calories, 16 g protein, 32 g carbs)

• 1 serving"Egg in a Hole" Peppers with Avocado Salsa

• 2 clementines

A.M. Sn ack (238calories, 7 g protein, 27 g carbs) (238calories, 7 g protein, 27 g carbs)

1 cup blueberries

20 unsalted almonds

Lunch (322calories, 22 g protein, 11 g carbs) (322calories, 22 g protein, 11 g carbs)

• 1 serving Salmon Salad-Stuffed Avocado P.M. Snack (78 calories, 1 g protein, 11 g carbs) (78 calories, 1 g protein, 11 g carbs)

• 1 Flourless Banana Chocolate Chip Mini Muffin

Dinner (389 calories, 10 g protein, 36 g carbs) (389 calories, 10 g protein, 36 g carbs) 1 servingWhiteBean Sage Cauliflower Gnocchi 2 cups mixed salad greens

1 Tbsp.Caesar Salad Dressing

¼ cup chopped tomato

¼ cup chopped cucumber 3 Tbsp. diced avocado

Toss salad greens with dressing, tomato, cucumber and avocado.

Daily Totals: 1,382 calories, 69 g fat, 32 g fiber, 103 g carbohydrates, 50 g protein, 1,565 mg sodium\sDay 2

To keep carbs low today , we included these sound flourless banana chocolate chip muffins made from oats, banana and eggs, and traded in zucchini noodles for regular pasta in tonight's supper. To make sure you are still getting adequate amounts of both carbohydrates and fiber, we filled in the rest of the day with nutrient-rich food sources like blackberries, edamame and a serving of entire wheat baguette at supper to sop up any of the scrumptious leftover juice from the scampi.

Br eakfast (352 calories, 27 g protein, 45 g carbs) (352 calories, 27 g protein, 45 g carbs)

2Flourless Banana Chocolate Chip Mini Muffins 1 cup raspberries

1 cup nonfat Greek yogurt

A.M. Snack (62calories, 2 g protein, 14 g carbs) (62calories, 2 g protein, 14 g carbs)

• 1 cup blackberries\sLunch (351 calories, 28 g protein, 14 g carbs) (351 calories, 28 g protein, 14 g carbs)

• 1 serving Chicken Satay Bowls with Spicy Peanut Sauce

P.M. Snack (200calories, 16 gprotein, 18 g carbs) (200calories, 16 gprotein, 18 g carbs)

• 1 cup shelled edamame, prepared with coarse salt and pepper, to taste

D inner (448 calories, 31 gprotein, 34 g carbs) (448 calories, 31 gprotein, 34 g carbs)

1 serving

Shrimp Scampi Zoodles 1 serving

Shrimp Scampi Zoodles

inch) cut whole-wheat baguette

1 tsp. olive oil to brush on baguette

Daily Totals: 1,414 calories, 105 g protein, 125 g carbs, 33 g fiber, 56 g fat,\s1,811 mg sodium

Day 3

Just a single cup of raspberries contains 8 grams of filling fiber with just 15 grams of carbs, which is why you'll see them often on this simple high- protein, lowcarb meal plan. High-fiber food varieties tend to be more filling than low-fiber foods, so you're likely to eat less and stay fulfilled longer, which is especially important when cutting calories to lose weight.

Breakfast (352 calories, 27 g protein, 45 g carbs) (352 calories, 27 g protein, 45 g carbs)

2Flourless Banana Chocolate Chip Mini Muffins 1 cup raspberries

1 cup non-fat Greek yogurt

A.M. Sn ack (262calories, 8 g protein, 25 g carbs)\s25 unsalted almonds

2 clementines\sLunch (351calories, 28 g protein, 14 gcarbs)\s• 1 serving Chicken Satay Bowls with Spicy Peanut Sauce

P.M. Sn ack (62 calories, 2 g protein, 14 g carbs) (62 calories, 2 g protein, 14 g carbs)

• 1 cup blackberries\sDinner (378calories, 32 gprotein, 31 g carbs) (378calories, 32 gprotein, 31 g carbs)

• 1 serving Pork Paprikash with Cauliflower "Rice"\s• 1 serving Roasted Fresh Green Beans

Daily Totals: 1,406 calories, 97 g protein, 128 g carbs, 43 g fiber, 62 g fat, 1,307 mg sodium\sDay 4

Moreover to being an incredible source of protein , which helps keep up with muscle mass while you're losing weight, salmon is a great source of omega-3 fatty acids, a fundamental fatty corrosive that you must get in your diet. Early research additionally shows that salmon eaters had lower fasting insulin levels, which can help keep your blood sugar in check and reduce your hazard for diabetes. Roasted salmon is served over low-carb veggie-licious kale and chickpeas-a healthy carb you can definitely still be eating, even when following a low-carb diet.

Br eakfast (269calories, 26 g protein, 33 g carbs) (269calories, 26 g protein, 33 g carbs)

1 cup nonfat plain Greek yogurt 1 cup raspberries

1 tsp. honey

1 Tbsp. chia seeds

A.M. Snack (262 calories, 18 gprotein, 32 g carbs) (262 calories, 18 gprotein, 32 g carbs) 1 cup shelled edamame, prepared with coarse salt and pepper, to taste 1 cup blackberries

Lunch (351calories, 28 g protein, 14 g carbs)\s• 1 serving Chicken Satay Bowls with Spicy Peanut Sauce

P.M. Snack (78calories, 1 g protein, 11 g carbs)\s• 1 Flourless Banana Chocolate Chip Mini Muffin

Dinner (447 calories, 37 g protein, 23 g carbs)\s• 1 serving Roasted Salmon with Smoky Chickpeas and Greens

Daily Totals: 1,407 calories, 111 g protein, 114 g carbs, 39 g fiber, 57 g fat, 1,505 mg sodium\sDay 5

Our high -protein weight-loss meal plan includes fiber-rich carbohydrates, similar to those from berries, white beans and broccoli. Supper tonight packs in 15 grams of protein, which helps you feel full as well as also may help with weight misfortune. In one study, researchers found that for every 10 grams of solvent fiber eaten over the course of a day, there was a corresponding 3.7 percent decrease in abdominal fat.

Breakfast (259calories, 15 g protein, 10 g carbs)\s• 1 serving Low-Carb Bacon and Broccoli Egg Burrito

A.M. Sn ack (218 calories, 7 g protein, 20 g carbs) (218 calories, 7 g protein, 20 g carbs)

1 cup raspberries

20 unsalted almonds

Lunch (351calories, 28 g protein, 14 gcarbs) (351calories, 28 g protein, 14 gcarbs)

• 1 servingChicken Satay Bowls with Spicy Peanut Sauce

P.M. Snack (129 calories, 6 g protein, 14 g carbs) (129 calories, 6 g protein, 14 g carbs) 1/4 cup hummus 4 celery stalks, cut into stalks

Dinner (442calories, 15 g protein, 50 g carbs) (442calories, 15 g protein, 50 g carbs)

• 1 serving Vegan Pesto Spaghetti Squash with Mushrooms and Sun-Dried Tomatoes

• 2/3 cup no-salt-added canned white beans, rinsed

Stir beans into an individual portion of the spaghetti squash and sauce.

Daily Totals: 1,407 calories, 111 g protein, 114 g carbs, 39 g fiber, 57 g fat, 1,505 mg sodium\sDay 6

Yes , you can still eat cheese and lose weight! String cheese is an extraordinary noontime snack, particularly when matched with fiber-rich raspberries. The combination of protein and fiber increases satisfaction and can lessen appetite at your next meal.

Br eakfast (269 calories, 26 g protein, 33 g carbs) (269 calories, 26 g protein, 33 g carbs)

1 cup nonfat plain Greek yogurt 1 cup raspberries

1 tsp. honey\s1 Tbsp. chia seeds

A.M. Snack (128 calories, 6 g protein, 22 g carbs) (128 calories, 6 g protein, 22 g carbs)

1 little apple

1 string cheese

Lunch (351 calories, 22 g protein, 14 gcarbs)\s• 1 serving Chicken Satay Bowls with Spicy Peanut Sauce

P.M. Sn ack (180calories, 6 g protein, 19 g carbs) (180calories, 6 g protein, 19 g carbs)

1 cup raspberries

15 unsalted almonds

Dinner (479calories, 25 gprotein, 28 g carbs) (479calories, 25 gprotein, 28 g carbs)

• 1 serving Taco Lettuce Wraps

• 1 serving Pineapple and Avocado Salad

Meal -Prep Tip: Save 1 serving of the Taco Lettuce Wraps to have for lunch on Day 7. When preparing the Pineapple and Avocado Salad, set aside 1/4 of an avocado and 1/2 cup pineapple before dressing with the vinaigrette to have for lunch on Day 7.

Daily Totals: 1,406 calories, 91 g protein, 115 g carbs, 39 g fiber, 7o g fat, 1,170 mg sodium\sDay 7

Lettuce takes the place of tortillas in our low -carb, gluten-free taco lettuce wraps. Stuffed with lean ground hamburger, jicama, avocado and salsa and a whopping 23 grams protein per serving, this lunch will keep you feeling full for hours.

Br eakfast (278 calories, 19 g protein, 22 g carbs)\s• 1 serving Spring Green Frittata\s• 1 cup raspberries

A.M. Snack (154calories, 5 g protein, 5 g carbs)\s• 20 unsalted almonds

Lunch (431 calories, 25 g protein, 28 g carbs) (431 calories, 25 g protein, 28 g carbs)

1 serving

Taco Lettuce Wraps 1/4 avocado, sliced\s1/2 cup cut pineapple

Combine avocado and pineapple with 1 tsp. lime juice and a squeeze of salt. P.M. Snack (62 calories, 2 g protein, 14 gcarbs) (62 calories, 2 g protein, 14 gcarbs)

• 1 cup blackberries

D inner (480calories, 33 g protein, 45 g carbs)\s• 1 serving Zucchini Lasagna\s••inch) slice whole-wheat baguette

Daily Totals: 1,405 calories, 84 g protein, 113 g carbs, 35 g fiber, 71 g fat, 1,685 mg sodium

HIGH PROTEIN LOWCARB DIET RECIPES\s1. Edamame Spaghetti With Kale CilantroPesto This bean pasta boasts just 22 grams of carbs per serving and keeps you full longer than other white and wheat pastas.

Serves: 4

Start to Finish: 18 minutes Prep: 10 minutes

Cook: 8 minutes

Ingredients:

1 cup of kale, tightly packed

1 cup of cilantro, firmly packed

1/4 cup of slivered almonds, toasted 1 garlic clove

1 serrano chile

1 tablespoon lime juice Dash of salt

1/4 cup of parmesan, grated 1/2 cup of olive oil

1handle ginger, sliced into shards Olive oil

2carrots, sliced into ribbons

1/4 cup of shredded coconut, toasted\s1box (8 oz) (8 oz) Explore Cuisine Edamame Spaghetti

Instructions:

1) Blend first seven ingredients in a food processor. Add cheese. Stream in olive oil. Sauté ginger in oil until crispy.

2) Boil 8 cups of water and pour in organic edamame spaghetti. Cook for 8 minutes. Drain. 3)Toss together edamame spaghetti with carrots and pesto. Top with ginger and toasted coconut. Nutrition Information (per serving): Calories: 471; Carbs: 29 g; Fat: 27 g; Protein: 29 g

2. Seared Peppercorn Ahi Tuna with ArugulaSalad This is an easy, light summer recipe that anybody can make and enjoy at home.

Skill level: Intermediat e Serves: 2 people

Start to Finish: 17 mins Prep: 5 mins

Cook: 12 mins

Ingr edients:

2(5 ounce) ahi tuna steaks 1 teaspoon kosher salt\s1/4 teaspoon cayenne pepper 2 tablespoons olive oil

1 tablespoon black peppercorn 1 teaspoon Zuzu sauce

Hannah An's Signature Garlic Lime Sauce

Instructions:\s1) Role the fish steaks in the salt, cayenne pepper, and dark peppercorn blend. Put olive oil in a skillet over medium-high heat.

2) Gently place the seasoned tuna in the skillet and cook to desired doneness. Cooking all sides evenly (1 1/2 minutes per side for rare). Slice tuna steaks in an upward direction in meager slices and top with Zuzu sauce.

3) Served with Fresh Arugula Salad and Tiato Leaf

Nutritional Information (per serving): Calories 302 ; Carbohydrate 2.9 g; Fat 9.2 g; Protein 51.3 g

3. Asparagus Wrapped in Chili Spiced Bacon

Asparagus wrapped in chili -spiced bacon is a simple dish that packs the flavor. It's a great snack option, consolidating vegetables and bacon to guarantee you're getting enough fat while skimping on the carbs.

Skill level: Beginner Serves: 4 servings

Start to Finish: 32 minutes Prep: 20 minutes Cook: 12 minutes

Ingredients:

1 teaspoon Chili Powder

1/2 teaspoon Sucralose Based Sweetener (Sugar Substitute) (Sugar Substitute) 4 slices bacon

24 spears Asparagus

Instructions:

1) Soak 16 wooden toothpicks in warm water for 20 minutes.

2) Preheat grill. Place a sheet of wax paper on a sheet container and set aside. Consolidate the bean stew powder and sugar substitute in a small bowl.

3) Cut bacon strips in half. Lay them on the sheet pan and dust with the chili powder mixture.

4) Wrap three asparagus lances together with one cut of bacon (with the dusted side facing towards the asparagus); securing each end with a toothpick. You ought to have 8 packets.

5) Grill uncovered over medium-low heat for 12 minutes turning halfway through or until bacon is crisp.

6) Discard toothpicks and serve immediately. Each serving is 2 wraps. Nutritional information

(per serving): Calories: 128; Net Carbs: 2.6 g; Fat: 10.2 g; Protein: 5g

4. Cauliflower Rice

This flavorful side dish will satisfy your "carb tooth" without any of the bloat. Skill level: Intermediate

Serves: 4-6

Start to Finish: 25 minutes Prep: 3 minutes

Cook: 22 minutes

Ingredients:

For Joes:

1 tablespoon olive oil

1 medium yellow onion, finely diced 2 garlic cloves, cleaved or minced

1 pound ground beef (or protein of decision: ground turkey, cooked lentils, or crumbled tempeh also work great) (or protein of decision: ground turkey, cooked lentils, or crumbled tempeh also work great)

1 to 2 teaspoons chile powder 2 teaspoons dried oregano

1 teaspoon sea salt 1/4 cup tomato paste 1/4 cup tomato paste\sounce) can tomato sauce

1 tablespoon Dijon mustard 1 cup water, optional

Garnishes: sliced toasted almonds, chopped fresh cilantro and/or parsley, optional

F or Rice:

1head cauliflower

2 tablespoons extravirgin olive oil 1 cup finely diced onion

2 cloves garlic, chopped or minced

Instructions:\s1) Start the rice by chopping the cauliflower florets and some of the stems into little pieces and pulse them in a food processor until they are the consistency of rice. Do not over-chop.

2) In a large skillet, heat 2 tablespoons of oil over low to medium heat and add the 1 cup onions and 2 cloves of garlic. Stir well and cook for 3 minutes.

3) Add the cauliflower rice from the food processor and cook for 10- 15minutes, till you feel it's fully cooked and flavors are well combined.

4) Meanwhile, heat the remaining tablespoon of oil in a separate container over medium-low heat.

5) Sauté the medium onion for around 10 minutes, until translucent. 6)Add the remaining garlic and sauté for 1 more minute.

7) Add protein of decision, chile powder, oregano, and salt and stir.

8) Add the tomato glue, tomato sauce, and mustard; mix and cook for 5 minutes.

9) Add water, up to a cup, as expected to make a sauce; mix and cook another 5 minutes, until protein is cooked through.

10) Serve promptly on top of cauliflower rice, and garnish as desired. Nutritional information (per serving): Calories: 321; Carbs: 13g; Fat: 23 g; Protein: 19 g

5. Spicy Turkey Lettuce Cups

This is a simple to -get ready, delicious and filling meal that has a low calorie count. If you like eating turkey burgers or tacos, these are the perfect low carb/low calorie substitute! They will fulfill your craving without sabotaging your weight loss.

Whisk together the heavy whipping cream and egg yolks in a little bowl until well combined.

Gently pour the egg mixture over the asparagus ingredients . Sprinkle with the crumbled goat cheese.

Bake at 350 degrees (F) for 25 minutes or until somewhat firm. Serve warm or chilled.

13. Baked Salmon with Creamy AvocadoSauce Tender pink salmon prepared in foil, then drizzled with zesty and creamy avocado sauce!

Prep Time10 minutes Cook Time20 minutes Total Time30 minutes Servings4

Ingr edients

4 little salmon fillets OR 2 enormous fillets (skin eliminated) (skin eliminated) 1/2 lemon Salt and pepper to taste

Avocado Sauce

1 huge ripe avocado

1/4 cup chopped cilantro

1 tablespoon fresh lemon juice 1 teaspoon garlic powder

1 teaspoon onion powder 1/2 teaspoon salt

Milk or water

Instructions

Preheat oven to 400 degrees. Line a baking sheet with a large piece of foil and oil lightly.

Place fillets in a solitary layer on pre -arranged baking sheet. Squeeze the lemon half to drizzle juice over the salmon fillets. Season both sides with salt and pepper to taste. Wrap the edges of the foil over the salmon fillets this helps to keep them damp! Bake for around 15-10 minutes or until flakey and tender.

While salmon is baking , prepare the sauce. Add avocado, cilantro, lime juice, garlic powder, onion powder, and salt to a blender or food processor and beat several times. Add milk or water 2-3 tablespoons at a period until mixture comes to a pourable consistency. Chill until ready to serve.

When salmon is completely cooked, drizzle with avocado sauce . If desired, serve salmon with additional chopped cilantro, new limes or lemons for squeezing, and rice.

14. Paleo Banana Bread Muffins

Light, moist and fluffy banana bread muffins are paleo, keto, sans gluten, lowcarb friendly. Time: 10 minutes

Cook Time: 15 minutes Total Time: 25 minutes Servings: muffins

Ingredients\s3 large eggs

2 cups mashed bananas 3-4 medium

1/2 cup almond butter peanut butter can additionally be used 1/4 cup spread olive oil can also be used

1 teaspoon vanilla

1/2 cup coconut flour almond flour can likewise be used 1 tablespoon cinnamon

1 teaspoon baking powder 1 teaspoon baking soda Pinch of ocean salt

1/2 cup chocolate chips discretionary and not included in nutritional facts

Instructions

Pre-heat oven to 350 degrees F. Grease or line 12 biscuit cups with liners; set aside.

Combine eggs, bananas, almond butter, butter, and vanilla in a large bowl . Speed until fully combined. Add the coconut flour, cinnamon, baking powder, baking pop, and squeeze of salt. Stir with a wooden spoon until fully combined.

Spoon hitter into biscuit tins, 3/4 full . Bake for 15-18 minutes or until golden. Cool for 10 minutes before removing from muffin tin. Store in refrigerator for up to 4 days.

15. HEMP-CRUSTED BAKED CHICKEN TENDER

Prep time: 15 MINUTES Cook time: 15 MINUTES Total time: 30 MINUTES Yield: 4-6 SERVINGS

These hemp-crusted baked chicken strips are simple to make, crispy, flavorful, and naturally

gluten-free.

INGREDIENTS

1/2 cup hemp seeds

1/2 cup ground almonds or almond meal 1 teaspoon garlic powder

1/2 teaspoon smoked paprika (or any paprika) (or any paprika) 1/2 teaspoon salt

1/4 teaspoon black pepper Pinch of cayenne pepper

1 1/2 pounds boneless, skinless chicken breasts, sliced into 1/4-inch thick strips

1/2 cup hemp seeds

2large eggs, whisked\sCooking spray (or you can also use olive oil in a Misto) (or you can also use olive oil in a Misto)

INSTRUCTIONS

Heat oven to 400 degrees F. Line a baking sheet with parchment paper.

In a medium bowl, whisk together hemp, ground almonds, garlic powder, paprika, salt, pepper and cayenne until evenly combined.

Set up your dipping stations in this order: (1) chicken strips (2) whisked eggs (3) hemp breading\s(4) parchment-lined baking sheet. Dip each chicken strip in the eggs until they are totally covered, then, at that point, give them a little shake to\slet any extra egg trickle off. Add the chicken strip to the hemp blend, and gently toss until the chicken strip is completely covered. Remove and transfer the chicken strip to the baking sheet. Repeat with remaining chicken. Give the chicken strips a good shot of cooking splash so that they are all delicately covered. Then bake for about 15-20 minutes, turningonce halfway through, until the chicken is cooked and no longer pink inside and the breading is golden.

Remove and serve warm with your desired plunging sauce.

16. ROASTED CAULIFLOWER WITH MARJORAM, PINE NUTS, GOLDEN RAISINS & LEMON

Ingredients

2.5 lbs. cauliflower, de-stemmed andslashed into 1 in. pieces 3 tablespoons olive oil 3tablespoons new marjoram leaves

1 teaspoon sea salt 2tablespoons butter 1 lemon, juice + zest

3garlic cloves, minced

1 leek, divided and meagerly sliced 1/4 cup pine nuts

1/3 cup golden raisins

1/4 cup roughly chopped parsley Sea salt to taste

Freshly ground pepper

Direction

Preheat oven to 375 degrees . Add cauliflower to a large baking sheet with olive oil, marjoram, sea salt and freshly ground pepper to taste. Broil for 25- 30 minutes or until browned and delicate. Add to serving bowl and set aside.

Add spread to a cast iron or sauté pan over medium low hotness . Add the zest of one lemon. Sauté until zest is fragrant, then add garlic and leeks. Stir often over low heat until leeks are relaxed, about 5-7 minutes. Add golden raisins until warm, then remove mixture and add to serving bowl.

Using the same pan, turn the heat up to medium and add pine nuts. Stir often for about 1-2 minutes or until pine nuts are browned and toasted. Remove from heat and add to serving bowl. Toss everything together with the juice of one lemon. Top with hacked parsley and season to taste. Serve immediately!

17. GRILLED HARISSA SHRIMP SKEWERS WITH BASIL OIL AND CILANTRO\sYIELD: 4-6 SERVINGS

My favorite way to serve these grilled shrimp sticks is with a generous drizzle of homemade basil oil simply basil leaves, olive oil, and ocean salt pureed in a blender and fresh cilantro leaves.

Prep time: 1 HOUR Cook time: 5 MINUTES

Total time: 1 HOUR 5 MINUTES

INGREDIENTS\sGRILLED HARISSA SHRIMP SKEWERS

1 lb wild crude unshelled shrimp (or 3/4 lb raw, shelled and de-veined shrimp) 1/4 cup Mina Mild Harissa, plus more for basting\skosher salt

Freshly ground black pepper Cooking oil spray

Fresh cilantro leaves

BASIL OIL

1 cup extra virgin olive oil

1 and 1/2 ounces of fresh basil leaves 1/4 teaspoon + 1/8 teaspoon kosher salt

INSTRUCTIONS

Marinate Shrimp: Shell and de-vein the shrimp and place in a medium bowl.

Throw with Mina mild harissa , cover the bowl with plastic wrap, and permit the shrimp to marinate in the refrigerator for 1 to 2 hours. Allow to rest at room temperature for 20-30 minutes before grilling.

Prepare Basil Oil : Place the oil, basil leaves, and salt in a blender container, and puree/mix until smooth. Place the oil in a little sealed shut container and store in the cooler until ready to use (oil can be put away in the ice chest for up to 3 weeks) (oil can be put away in the ice chest for up to 3 weeks).

Using small wooden sticks (soak the skewers in water if using on an outdoor grill), thread 3-4 shrimp on each skewer, running the skewer through the neck and once near the tail (see photographs above) (see photographs above). Lightly season the shrimp with salt and pepper. Place a limited quantity (2-3 tablespoons) of Mina gentle harissa in a small bowl (do not use the marinade for this step) for treating and set aside.

Heat a large (10 to 12 -inch) non-stick grill pan over medium-high heat, and spray with cooking oil. Lay the shrimp skewers in the grill pan (do not over crowd the pan) and barbecue on for 2-3 minutes on each side brushing the shrimp with additional harissa as you grill them or until the shrimp are opaque and cooked through

Drizzle the shrimp sticks with basil oil and embellish with fresh cilantro leaves. Serve immediately.

18. Chicken Avocado Burgers

Prep Time 10 mins Cook Time 15 mins Total Time 25 mins

A new twist on a Chicken Avocado Burger! Mix cubed avocado directly into your ground chicken for a super kicked up avocado flavor!

Course: Main Course Cuisine: American Servings: 4 Burger

Ingr edients

1 pound ground chicken\s1 enormous ripe avocado cut into chunks 1 clove chopped of garlic 1/3 cup Panko crumbs or Almond

1 minced Poblano or Jalapeño pepper optional however recommended 1/2 teaspoon salt

1/4 teaspoon pepper

In structions

Add all ingredients to a large bowl and toss gently. Shape into wanted size patties.

. 5 minutes on each side on an indoor grill pan or an outside grill at medium heat or until the internal temperature comes to 165 degrees.

19. Broccoli Crust Pizza

Prep Time: 5 minutes Cook Time: 20 minutes Total Time: 25 minutes

Ingredients Broccoli Crust:\s1 little head of broccoli about 2-3 cups riced 2 eggs

1/4 cup parmesan cheddar 1/4 cup mozzarella cheddar 1/4 teaspoon salt 1/4 teaspoon pepper\s1/2 teaspoon italian seasoning optional

Toppings

1/4 cup pizza sauce 1 cup cheese Veggies optional

Instructions

Pre-heat oven to 400 degrees F. Line a baking sheet with parchment paper (exceptionally recommend) or oil with oil; set aside.

Process the broccoli in a food processor or shred with a cheese grater until the broccoli is the equivalent consistency as rice.

Place broccoli in an enormous bowl , cover with plastic wrap and micorwave cover with plastic wrap and micorwave 2 minute or until it is steamed. Cool for at least one minute then pour broccoli on a spotless washcloth and squeeze as much fluid as you can out of the broccoli until you are left with a dry ball of broccoli.

In an enormous bowl , consolidate the broccoli, eggs, cheeses, and seasoning with a spoon until completely combined. Pour combinationinto the pre-lined baking sheet and shape into a pizza crust, 1/2 inch thick. Heat for 10-12 minutes or until outside layer is gently browned. Remove from the broiler and add the pizza sauce and cheese. At this point feel free to add desired garnishes (veggies or meat) (veggies or meat). Return to the oven and bake for an additional Return to the oven and bake for an additional 12 minutes or until the cheese is fully softened. Cool for no less than 5 minutes before cutting.

20. Philly Cheese Steak ZucchiniBoats

All the flavors of the classic Philly Cheesesteak sandwich without loads of carbs. Made in zucchini boats instead of heavy bread yet still totally delicious!

Servings: 4

Prep Time 15 minutes Cook Time 25 minutes Total Time 40 minutes

Ingr edients

4 medium/large wide zucchini (2 1/2 lbs) 3 Tbsp olive oil, divided

1 large yellow onion, cut into short pieces 8 little button mushrooms (6 oz), sliced 1 large red or green bell pepper, hacked into short slices (or 1/2 of a red 1/2 of a green)

2 garlic cloves, minced

3/4 lb sliced flimsy deli roast beef, cleaved into small pieces Salt and freshly ground black pepper

1 1/2 Tbsp water or meat broth 1 1/4 cups shredded provolone\scheddar Chopped fresh parsley, for serving

Instructions

Preheat broiler to 400 degrees . Using a spoon, scoop focuses from zucchini to make boats while leaving a 1/4-inch rim (hold focuses for another utilization) (hold focuses for another utilization). Brush the two sides of zucchini with 1 Tbsp of the olive oil and season gently with salt. Place in two baking pans (I used a 13 by 9 and 8 by 8). (I used a 13 by 9 and 8 by 8). Bake in preheated oven 20 25 minutes until almost tender. Meanwhile, heat 1 Tbsp olive oil in a large non-stick skillet over medium- high heat. Add onion and saute 5 minutes, then, at that point, add another 1/2 Tbsp olive oil and mushrooms and saute 5 minutes longer.

Push veggies to one side of pan then add staying 1/2 Tbsp olive oil to opposite side, add bell pepper and garlic and saute until tender, about 3 minutes. Add in roast beef, season with salt and pepper to taste then stir in water and cook until warmed, about 30 seconds.

Fill roasted zucchini with roast hamburger mixture . Sprinkle top evenly with cheddar. Get back to broiler and bake about 5 minutes longer, or until cheddar has melted. Serve warm garnished with parsley (fyi these are easier to just pick up and eat by hand like a sandwich) (fyi these are easier to just pick up and eat by hand like a sandwich).

*You can likewise make these into the classic Philly Cheese Steak Sandwiches by using 4 hoagie rolls in place of the zucchini and upping the broil beef to 1 lb.

21. Cobb Salad Recipe

Prep Time 20 mins Total Time 20 mins

Cobb Salad Recipe This classic American main-dish salad is loaded with chicken, avocado, sweet tomatoes, crunchy bacon, blue cheese, and eggs, all beat with an eased up blue cheddar dressing.

Course: Salad Cuisine: American Servings: 4\sCalories: 389 kcal

Ingredients\sFOR THE DRESSING

3/4-cup non-fat plain yogurt

1 tablespoon extra virgin olive oil 1 teaspoon white vinegar 1teaspoon Dijon mustard

2tablespoons reduced fat disintegrated blue cheese Salt and new ground pepper, to taste

FOR THE SALAD

10 cups blended salad greens

8 ounces destroyed cooked chicken breast

4 slices turkey bacon, cooked to a desired freshness and crumbled 3 enormous hard boiled eggs, sliced\s1 cup cherry tomatoes, split 1 avocado, sliced\s1/2 cup reduced fat crumbled blue cheese

Instructions

Prepare the dressing by combining all ingredients in a mixing bowl; whisk together until thoroughly joined. Set aside.

Arrange salad greens on an enormous plate.

Arrange chicken, bacon, egg, tomatoes, avocado, and blue cheese on top of the salad greens.

Drizzle the salad with previously prepared dressing . Serve.

TO MAKE THE WRAPS (OPTIONAL) (OPTIONAL)

Heat lowcarb flour tortilla wraps in the microwave.

Spread about 2 tablespoons of the dressing over each flour tortilla. Place a few salad greens in the middle of the flour tortilla.

Add some chicken, a bit of disintegrated bacon, couple cuts of eggs, some tomatoes, a slice of avocado, and sprinkle with disintegrated blue cheese. Roll it up tightly; cut in half and serve.

22. Colorful Beet Salad with Carrot, Quinoa & Spinach Prep Time: 30 mins Cook Time: 15 mins Total\sTime: 45 minutes Yield: 2\sto 4 salads

INGREDIENTS

Salad

½ cup uncooked quinoa, rinsed 1 cup frozen natural edamame

⅓ cup slivered almonds or pepitas (green pumpkin seeds) (green pumpkin seeds) 1 medium crude beet, peeled\s1 medium-to-large carrot (or 1 additional medium beet), stripped 2 cups packed baby spinach or arugula, generally chopped

1 avocado, cubed Vinaigrette

3 tablespoons apple cider vinegar 2 tablespoons lime juice

2 tablespoons olive oil

1tablespoon slashed fresh mint or cilantro 2tablespoons honey or maple syrup or agave nectar

½ to 1 teaspoon Dijon mustard, to taste\s¼ teaspoon salt

Freshly ground black pepper, to taste\sINSTRUCTIONS

To cook the quinoa : First, flush the quinoa in a fine mesh colander under running water for a minute or two. In a medium-sized pot, consolidate the flushed quinoa and 1 cup water. Bring the blend to a gentle boil, then cover the pot, reduce heat to a simmer and cook for 15 minutes.

Eliminate the quinoa from heat and let it rest, still covered, for 5 minutes. Uncover the pot, drain off any abundance water and cushion the quinoa with a fork. Set it aside to cool.

To cook the edamame: Bring a pot of water to bubble, then add the frozen edamame and cook just until the beans are warmed through, around 5 minutes. Channel and set aside.

To toast the almonds or pepitas : In a little skillet over medium heat, toast the almonds or pepitas, stirring frequently, until they are fragrant and starting to become brilliant on the edges, about 5 minutes. Transfer to an enormous serving bowl to cool.

To prepare the beet(s) and/or carrot : First of all, feel free to just chop them as finely as possible utilizing a sharp chef's blade OR mesh them on a box grater. Assuming you have a spiralizer, you can spiralize them using blade C, cleave the ribbons into small pieces using a sharp chef's blade. Ifyou have a mandolineand juliennepeeler (this is apain), use the mandoline to julienne the beet and use a julienne peeler to julienne the carrot, then chop the ribbons into small pieces using a sharp chef's knife.

To prepare the vinaigrette: Whisk together all of the fixings until emulsified.

To assemble the salad: In your enormous serving bowl, combine the toasted almonds/pepitas, cooked edamame, prepared beet(s) and/or carrot, generally hacked spinach/arugula (see note above about leftovers), cubed avocado and cooked quinoa.

Finally, drizzle dressing over the mixture (you might not need all of it) and delicately throw to combine. You'll end up with a pink salad if you throw it truly well! Season to taste with salt (up to an additional ¼ teaspoon) and black pepper. Serve.

23. CRISPY SLOW COOKER CARNITAS

Crispy, delicate, falling apart pork covered in so much flavour, you will not be able to put your forks down!

INGREDIENTS

4 pounds (2 kg) boneless pork shoulder (pork butt), trimmed of any abundance fat 1 tablespoon olive oil

1 tablespoon dried oregano 1 tablespoon ground cumin

1 tablespoon paprika (sweet or smokey) (sweet or smokey)

1 1/2 2 tablespoons ocean salt pieces OR 1 tablespoon table salt (change to your tastes) (change to your tastes) 1 teaspoon freshly ground black pepper

2 tablespoons brown sugar 1 onion, coarsely chopped

6 large cloves garlic, cut in half

1jalapeno, deseeded and ribs removed, hacked jalapeno, deseeded and ribs removed, hacked ounce (410g) (410g) can crushed tomatoes

Juice from 2 limes (1/4 cup lime juice)

2ancho chiles (poblano peppers), deseeded, ribs eliminated and sliced INSTRUCTIONS Slow Cooker Method:

Rinse and dry the pork shoulder with paper towel . Place the pork in slow cooker bowl and add in the oil, oregano, cumin, paprika, salt, pepper and brown sugar on the pork. Rub seasoning all over pork; top with the onion, garlic, and jalapeno.

Add in the tomatoes and press the lime juices over the pork. Mix everything together until well combined.

Cover and cook on low for 8 to 10 hours or on high 4 to 5 hours . Once the meat is fork tender and falling apart, eliminate from slow cooker and allow to cool slightly before pulling apart with 2 forks.

Place the carnitas (destroyed meat) onto a baking tray; drizzle with sauce from the slow cooker; add the ancho chiles (poblano peppers) and permit to grill/broil in a preheated broiler on medium-high settings until brilliant and crispy. On the other hand, place destroyed pork into a skillet and fry until crispy with the chile cuts over medium-high heat.

Oven Method:\sPreheat broiler to 120°C | 250°F. Place an oven rack in the lower-middle part of your oven.

Coat pork in spices and sauces as above . Put the pork in a roasting container and cover skillet firmly with foil. Heat for around 6-8 hours, or until falling apart, seasoning it in it's own juices after three hours or so. Add in the ancho pepper strips during the last hour of roasting (if including) (if including).

Shred as above.

24. SUN DRIED TOMATO CHEESY MEATBALLS

Tender and juicy meatballs spiked with sun dried tomato pieces, garlic and new herbs, fried and simmered in a straightforward tomato sauce with so much cheese.

INGREDIENTS

Meatballs:

500 g hamburger mince

500 g pork mince (or utilize additional meat mince) (or utilize additional meat mince) 1 egg, lightly whisked

1/2cup almond flour (or 1/3 cup breadcrumbs if not following low carb) 150 g semi-dried tomatoes, drained and oil reserved 1/2 cup ground Parmesan cheese

4 cloves garlic, crushed

4 table spoons tomato paste

1 tablespoon fresh cleaved oregano 1 tablespoon new chopped basil 1tablespoon oil

Salt to taste (around 1 tablespoon) (around 1 tablespoon) and pepper

S auce:\sheld Sun Dried Tomato oil\s2x 420g jars tomato pasta sauce (or tomato soup) (or tomato soup)

180 g large bocconcini balls (6 large balls the size of golf balls), sliced

INSTRUCTIONS

Combine mince, egg and almond flour, tomatoes drained of oi l (hold oil), cheese, garlic, paste, oregano and basil in a bowl. Season with salt and pepper. Shape into 12 meatballs (I utilized full palm sized meat mixture) (I utilized full palm sized meat mixture).

Heat oil in a non stick oven proof pan or cast iron skillet over medium heat . Cook meatballs, in clusters for 3 to 4 minutes while occasionally turning to brown on all sides.

Heat reserved semi-dried tomatoes oil in pan. Add the tomato sauce (or soup) (or soup). Cook, stirring, for 2 minutes.

Return meatballs to pan; bring to the boil; reduce heat to low and allow to simmer, covered for 15-20 minutes or until meatballs have cooked through and sauce has thickened.

Meanwhile, preheat oven to grill (or broil) settings on medium heat halfway through cooking time. When meatballs are ready, arrange the bocconcini slices over the meatballs and place pan into the oven. Grill/broil until cheddar hasmelted.

25. CREAMY HONEY MUSTARD CHICKEN WITH CRISPY BACON

A deliciously Creamy Honey Mustard Chicken with firm bacon pieces will become your new favourite supper, with dairy free options!

PREP: 10 MINS

COOK: 15 MINS

TOTAL: 25 MINS

SERVES: 5

INGREDIENTS

1/3 cup honey

3 level tablespoons whole grain mustard

1 1/2 tablespoons minced garlic, (or 3-4 cloves squashed garlic) (or 3-4 cloves squashed garlic) 1 tablespoon olive oil

Salt to season

5 skinless and boneless chicken bosoms (or chicken thighs) (or chicken thighs)

1/2 cup diced bacon, trimmed of skin and fat (I utilized 4 little bacon rashers) (I utilized 4 little bacon rashers)

1/3 cup cream (light or reduced fat) *SEE NOTES FOR SUBSTITUTION OPTIONS 1 cup milk (skim, 2 percent or full fat -almond milk may be utilized for a dairy free option) (skim, 2 percent or full fat -almond milk may be utilized for a dairy free option)

1 teaspoon cornstarch (corn flour) mixed with 1 tablespoon water 2 tablespoon chopped new parsley

INSTRUCTIONS

In a large, shallow dish, consolidate the honey, mustard, garlic, oil and salt to taste (not an excess of salt if presenting with bacon as the bacon will add a salty flavour when served) (not an excess of salt if presenting with bacon as the bacon will add a salty flavour when served). Coat chicken equitably in the sauce. Set aside.

Heat a nonstick pan (or skillet) over medium heat . Fry bacon until crispy; transfer to a plate. To the same skillet, sear chicken fillets on each side in the oil left over from the bacon until just starting to brown (around 3 minutes per side not completely cooked through as we will complete them in the sauce) (around 3 minutes per side not completely cooked through as we will complete them in the sauce). Add any remaining honey mustard sauce into the pan along with the cream and milk. Bring to a stew while stirring occasionally to mix the favours through the sauce (about 3 minutes), until the chicken is cooked through. Transfer the chicken to a warm plate.

Pour the cornstarch mixture into the centre of the pan, mixing it through the sauce until it thickens. Place chicken back into the pan; cover with the sauce. Top with the bacon and garnish with parsley.

Serve over steamed/roasted vegetables for lower cal options. Also extraordinary with pasta, rice or pounded potatoes!

26. CREAMY HONEY MUSTARD CHICKEN WITH CRISPY BACON

A deliciously Creamy Honey Mustard Chicken with firm bacon pieces will become your new favourite dinner, with dairy free options!

PREP: 10 MINS COOK: 15 MINS TOTAL: 25 MINS SERVES: 5

INGREDIENTS

1/3 cup honey

3 level tablespoons entire grain mustard

1 1/2 tablespoons minced garlic, (or 3-4 cloves squashed garlic) (or 3-4 cloves squashed garlic) 1 tablespoon olive oil

Salt to season

5 skinless and boneless chicken breasts (or chicken thighs) (or chicken thighs)

1/2 cup diced bacon, managed of rind and fat (I utilized 4 small bacon rashers) (I utilized 4 small bacon rashers) 1/3 cup cream (light or reduced fat) (light or reduced fat) *SEE NOTES FOR SUBSTITUTION OPTIONS

1 cup milk (skim, 2 percent or full fat -almond milk may be used for a dairy free option) (skim, 2 percent or full fat - almond milk may be used for a dairy free option)

1 teaspoon cornstarch (corn flour) mixed with 1 tablespoon water 2 tablespoon chopped new parsley

INSTRUCTIONS

In a large, shallow dish, join the honey, mustard, garlic, oil and salt to taste (not too much salt if serving with bacon as the bacon will add a salty flavor when served) (not too much salt if serving with bacon as the bacon will add a salty flavor when served). Coat chicken evenly in the sauce. Set aside.

Heat a nonstick dish (or skillet) over medium heat . Fry bacon until crispy; transfer to a plate. To the same pan, sear chicken fillets on each side in the oil left over from the bacon until just beginning to brown (around 3 minutes per side not totally cooked through as we will finish them in the sauce) (around 3 minutes per side not totally cooked through as we will finish them in the sauce).

Add any remaining honey mustard sauce into the dish along with the cream and milk. Bring to a stew while stirring sometimes to mix the favors through the sauce (about 3 minutes), until the chicken is cooked through. Transfer the chicken to a warm plate.

Pour the cornstarch mixture into the focus of the pan, mixing it through the sauce until it thickens. Place chicken back into the pan; cover with the sauce. Top with the bacon and decorate with parsley.

Serve over steamed/broiled vegetables for lower cal choices. Likewise extraordinary with pasta, rice or squashed potatoes!

27. CHICKEN AND ASPARAGUS LEMON STIR FRY PREP TIME: 5 mins COOK TIME: 25 mins

TOTAL TIME: 30 mins YIELD: 4 SERVING

This speedy chicken and asparagus pan sear made with chicken breast, fresh lemon, garlic and ginger is the perfect fast weeknight dish.

INGREDIENTS

11/2 pounds skinless chicken breast, cut into 1-inch cubes Kosher salt, to taste

1/2 cup decreased sodium chicken broth\s2tablespoons reduced-sodium shoyu or soy sauce, Coconut aminos for GF, W30

2 teaspoons cornstarch, arrowroot powder or custard starch for whole30 2 tablespoons water 1 tbsp canola or grapeseed oil, divided\s1 bunch asparagus, closes trimmed, cut into 2-inch pieces 6 cloves garlic, chopped\s1 tbsp fresh ginger

3 tablespoons new lemon juice Fresh dark pepper, to taste

INSTRUCTIONS

Lightly season the chicken with salt.

In a little bowl, combine chicken broth and soy sauce.

In a moment small bowl combine the cornstarch and water and mix well to combine.

Heat a large non -stick wok over medium-high heat, when hot add 1 teaspoon of the oil, then add the asparagus and cook until tender-crisp, about 3 to 4 minutes.

Add the garlic and ginger and cook until golden, around 1 minute . Set to the side. Increase the heat to high, then add 1 teaspoon of oil and half of the chicken\sand cook until browned and cooked through, about 4 minutes on each side.

Remove and set aside and repeat with the leftover oil and chicken. Set aside.

Add the soy sauce combination; bring to a bubble and cook around 1-1/2 minutes.

Add lemon juice and cornstarch mixture and stir well, when it stews return the chicken and asparagus to the wok and mix well, remove from heat and serve.

28. CREAMY SUNDRIED TOMATO + PARMESAN CHICKEN ZOODLES

Sundried tomatoes and garlic and parmesan cheddar infused in a cream based sauce, enveloping crispy, golden pan fried chicken tenders and zoodles for the craziest low carb solace food.

PREP: 15 MINS

COOK: 15 MINS

TOTAL: 30 MINS

SERVES: 6

INGREDIENTS

1 tablespoon butter\s700 g | 1 1/2 lb skinless chicken thigh fillets , cut into strips

120 g | 4oz fresh semi-dried tomato strips in oil, chopped *See Notes 100 g | 3.5oz jarred sun dried tomatoes in oil, chopped\s4 cloves garlic, peeled and crushed

300 ml |

1 1/4 cup thickened cream, reduced fat or full fat (or half and half) (or half and half) 1 cup shaved Parmesan cheese

Salt to taste

Dried basil seasoning Red chilli flakes

2 enormous Zucchini (or summer squash), made into Zoodles (use a vegetable grater if you don't have a Zoodle grater)

INSTRUCTIONS

Heat the margarine in a pan/skillet over medium high heat . Add the chicken strips and sprinkle with salt. Sauté until the chicken is golden browned on all sides and cooked through.

Add both semi -dried and sun dried tomatoes with 1 tablespoon of the oil from the jar (discretionary however adds extra flavour), and add the garlic; sauté until fragrant. (While the chicken is searing, set up your Zoodles with a Zoodle maker OR with a normal vegetable peeler.)

Lower heat, add the cream and the Parmesan cheddar; simmer while mixing until the cheddar has melted through. Sprinkle over salt, basil and red chilli flakes to your taste.

Stir through the Zoodles and continue to simmer until the zoodles have softened to your liking (around 5-8 minutes) and serve.

Gumbo with shrimp and sausage (nineteenth) 30 minute prep 1 hr 30 min to prepare

8 servings (approximately).

509 cals

INGREDIENTS

1 pound raw shrimp, peeled and deveined 4 smoked Andouille sausage links (approximately 12 ounces) 2 red and orange bell peppers, chopped 1 yellow onion, chopped

20 carrots, baby-cut (about 1 cup) 28 oz. squashed tomatoes 5 scallions, sliced 4 cup broth de poulet

To prepare the roux, combine the following ingredients in a blender and blend until smooth.

all-purpose flour, 1/2 cup 1 teaspoon of butter

Canola oil (1/4 cup)

F or a cajun seasoning mixture:

2 tsp garlic powder 1 tsp dried thyme paprika, 2 tblsp.

1 teaspoon dry minced onion 2 teaspoons salt 1 teaspoon cayenne pepper

1 tsp chili powder

INSTRUCTIONS

To make the cajun seasoning, combine all of the following ingredients in a small mixing bowl. In a small mixing bowl, combine and mix the cajun fixings. Remove the item from circulation.

To make the roux, combine all of the ingredients in a mixing bowl and whisk In a large pot or dutch oven (at least 5 quarts), heat the canola oil over medium heat. Combine the flour and the spread. Cook, stirring constantly, for about 15 minutes, or until the roux turns a dull caramel shade.

Add the bell peppers, onions, and carrots to the pot with the roux to cook. Stir in the roux until it's completely mixed in. Cook for 10 minutes, stirring occasionally, until the vegetables have softened and become fragrant.

Add liquids and spices to the pot to simmer: Combine the squashed tomatoes (including liquid), chicken broth, and salt and pepper in a large mixing bowl.

to the equivalent pot, add the scallions and cajun seasoning Bring to a boil, then reduce to a medium heat and allow to simmer. Allow for 1 hour of simmering time after covering with a lid.

Uncover the pot and add shrimp and hotdog. In the same pot, combine the shrimp and wiener. Allow about 5 minutes for the shrimp to become opaque and cooked. Remove the pan from the heat and serve immediately with rice.

Soup with No Tortillas (no tortilla) (no tortillas) (no tortillas) (no tortillas

Remove the seeds from the jalapeos before dicing them if you don't like spicy foods.

INGREDIENTS

1 tbsp. ghee (clarified butter) (explained butter) 1 large, diced yellow onion 6 peeled and minced garlic cloves

2 diced new jalapeos (and cultivated, if you wish) chicken stock (two quarts) Fire-roasted tomatoes, 11 oz.

1 cooked and diced pound of chicken breast a cup of chopped fresh cilantro two limes (juice)

To serve, garnish with avocado slices, lime pinwheels, or fresh cilantro minced.

DIRECTIONS

Ghee should be heated over medium heat in a Dutch stove or soup pot. Cook for 4 to 6 minutes, or until onions are clear.

Garlic and jalapeo peppers should be added at this point. 1–2 minutes, or until fragrant Bring the chicken stock and tomatoes to a medium boil, then reduce to a low heat and cook for 3–5 minutes.

Stir in the cooked chicken, cilantro, and lime juice until everything is well combined. Enjoy the soup with whatever garnish you like!

31. CILANTRO AND LIME CHICKEN AND AVOCADO SALAD

4 SERVINGS YIELDS

15 MINUTES FOR PREPARE 15 MINUTES TOTAL WORK TIME

The flavors in this Low-Carb Chicken and Avocado Salad with Lime and Cilantro are superb.

INGREDIENTS

2 c. cooked chicken, shredded into huge chunks 2 t fresh lime juice 2 medium avocados, diced to taste with salt

1 cup green onion, thinly sliced

fresh cilantro, finely chopped (or chop it more coarsely if you prefer)

INSTRUCTIONS

Shred the chicken into large chunks until you have 2 cups.

Avocados should be diced into medium-sized pieces, then mixed with 1 tablespoon lime juice and salt to taste.

Green onion, thinly sliced, and cilantro, finely chopped To make the dressing, whisk together 1 tablespoon mayonnaise and 1 teaspoon lime juice.

Place the chicken in a large mixing bowl that can accommodate all of the salad ingredients. Toss in the sliced green onions and the dressing until the chicken is thoroughly coated.

In the bottom of the bowl, combine the avocado and any lime juice with the chicken and toss tenderly.

Then, just barely combine the chopped cilantro with the salad.

Serve right away or chill until ready to serve. This could be served in pita bread, sandwich bread, or lettuce cups, but we just ate it as a salad.

I'm sure it'll keep in the fridge for a few days, but I didn't have any when I made it!

32. EGG CUPS WITH CAULIFLOWER HASH 15 MINUTES TO PREPARE AND 20 MINUTES TO COOK

35 MINUTES TOTAL

12 PARTS

INGREDIENTS

1 cauliflower head, cut into florets with the stalk and leaves removed furthermore 1 whisked large egg

cheddar cheese, 1/2 cup (or Mozzarella) Parmesan cheese, grated

Parmesan cheese, grated salt, 1 teaspoon (to your tastes) cayenne (optional -to taste)

garlic powder (1/2 teaspoon) (or 1 teaspoon onion powder) 12 medium-sized eggs, 12 small eggs

INSTRUCTIONS

Preheat the oven to 230°C | 350°F. Lightly spray a 12-hole muffin tin with cooking oil splash (or butter) and set aside.

Pulse the cauliflower in two clumps for 30 – 50 seconds, or until a fine 'rice' forms. If there are a few larger pieces in there, that's fine. (If you process the cauliflower too much, it will turn into a raw puree.)

In a microwave-safe bowl, measure out 3 cups (480g or 17oz) cauliflower rice and heat for about 8 minutes or until soft. Alternatively, lightly steam over a pot of boiling water or in a vegetable steamer until soft. Eliminate and allow to cool for a good 5 minutes before handling.

Using paper towels , an old tea towel or a cheesecloth, squeeze out as much liquid as you can until hardly any liquid can be squeezed out. (It's simpler to wrap the cauliflower in the towel (or cloth) and squeeze it into a ball over the sink. Less mess)

Transfer back into your bowl (make sure there's no liquid in it), and add the whisked egg, cheeses, salt and garlic powder.

Divide the blend into each muffin hole and firmly press them with your fingertips to create a 'nest' or cup.

Bake for about 15 -20 minutes or until the cheddar has softened, the cups are brilliant and the edges are browned. Remove from the oven; break the eggs into each cup; season with salt and pepper; return to the oven and bake for an into each cup; season with salt and pepper; return to the oven and bake for a 15 minutes, or until the whites are set and the yolks are cooked to your liking.

Allow them to cool for 5 minutes before handling them , or they may fall apart. Lightly slide a blade around the sides of each cup. Utilizing a fork, delicately lift one side first to make sure they're not sticking to the bottom, and lift out of the pan.

Garnish with red chilli flakes and parsley (discretionary) or leave as is.

33. ORANGE CHICKEN LETTUCE WRAPS

Prep time: 5 MINS Cook time: 15 MINS Total time: 20 MINS

Easy to make, light and healthy orange chicken lettuce wraps! The ground chicken tastes just like a healthier form of orange chicken and being in lettuce wraps means it's a low carb, high protein, filling meal for lunch or dinner.

INGREDIENTS:

ORANGE CHICKEN SAUCE:

1/2 cup orange juice 1tablespoons orange zest 2 tablespoons soy sauce

2tablespoons apple cider vinegar 1/4 cup brown sugar

1 teaspoon garlic, minced

1/2 teaspoon EACH ground ginger AND red pepper flakes 2 tablespoons water AND 1/2 tablespoons cornstarch

CHICKEN FILLING:

1 tablespoon oil

1 pound ground chicken (turkey or beef works too) (turkey or beef works too) 2 teaspoons garlic, minced

1 (10. 5 ounce) can mandarin oranges (new dollface slices work too) (new dollface slices work too) cleaved scallions, lettuce leaves AND toasted sesame seeds for decorating ORANGE CHICKEN SAUCE: Combine the

elements for the sauce in an artisan jar, give it a few good shakes until all the ingredients are blended. Pour the sauce into a small pan and heat over medium high heat. When the sauce begins to stew, lower the heat and allow to cook for an extra 1-2 minutes. You need the sauce to be thick enough to coat the back of a spoon. Remove from stove, allow to cool.

CHICKEN FILLING: Heat the oil in a large skillet over medium-high heat. Add the ground chicken and break down any lumps with a wooden spoon, then add the garlic and let the chicken cook for 5-7 minutes or until it cooks all the way through. Sprinkle the chicken with the prepared sauce. Let cook for 1-2 minutes. Adjust with salt and pepper to taste. Allow the filling to cool for several minutes before filling lettuce leaves. Top with mandarin orange cuts and toasted sesame seeds.

34. GARLIC BUTTER BAKED SALMON IN FOIL Prep time: 5 MINS Cook time: 20 MINS

Total time: 25 MINS

Garlic spread baked salmon in no time at all! Start with a straightforward lemon garlic margarine sauce that's super fancy yet also truly easy to make then we just pour this on top of a filet of salmon and prepare it off in the oven wrapped in foil. The salmon is flakey and delicate this way, and the garlic butter flavor is out of this world!

INGREDIENTS:\s1¼ pound sockeye or coho salmon (ideally wild caught)* 2 tablespoons EACH: lemon juice AND cold butter, cubed 2cloves garlic, minced\s½ teaspoon salt

¼ teaspoon EACH: Italian seasoning, red pepper chips AND black pepper 1 tablespoon hacked parsley, for embellishing (optional) (optional)

PREP: Position a rack in the center of the oven and preheat the oven to 375°F.

SAUCE: In a saucepan over medium heat, combine the lemon juice and minced garlic, permit the lemon juice to reduce to 1 tablespoon. Add in 1 tablespoon of butter, remove pan from heat and swirl so the butter begins to melt. Place back on the hotness for a few seconds, removed and continue to swirl until butter totally melts. Repeat with second tablespoon of butter. When butter is completely liquefied, add the Italian preparing, red pepper flakes, salt and pepper. Then, remove sauce from stove.

BAKE: Place the salmon filet in a piece of foil large enough to overlap over and seal. Utilizing a brush or spoon, brush the salmon with the garlic spread sauce. Cover with foil so that all sides are properly closed so the sauce doesn't leak. Bake the salmon for 12-14 minutes or until mostly firm to the touch. Open the foil and allow the fish to cook under the oven for 2-3 minutes, keeping an eye on it so the fish doesn't consume. Remove from oven, top with parsley. Serve immediately.

35. CHICKEN AVOCADO CAPRESE SALAD

Balsamic Chicken Avocado Caprese Salad is a fast and simple meal in a plate of mixed greens! Seared chicken, fresh mozzarella and tomato parts, creamy avocado cuts and shredded basil

leaves are sprinkled with an unimaginable balsamic dressing that doubles as a marinade for the ultimate salad!

PREP: 5 MINS

COOK: 15 MINS

TOTAL: 20 MINS

SERVES: 4

INGREDIENTS

Marinade/Dressing:\s1/4 cup (60 mL) (60 mL) balsamic vinegar 2 tablespoons (30 mL) olive oil

2 teaspoons brown sugar 1 teaspoon minced garlic 1 teaspoon dried basil

1 teaspoon salt

S alad:\s4chicken thigh fillets, skin removed (no bone)*\s5cups Romaine, (or cos) lettuce leaves, washed and dried 1 avocado, sliced\s1 cup cherry or grape tomatoes, sliced

1/2 cup mini mozzarella/bocconcini cheddar balls 1/4 cup basil leaves, thinly sliced

Salt and pepper, to season

INSTRUCTIONS

Whisk marinade ingredients together to combine . Place chicken into a shallow dish; pour 4 tablespoons of the dressing/marinade onto the chicken and stir around to equally coat chicken. Reserve the untouched marinade to use as a dressing.

Heat about one teaspoon of oil in a large grill dish or skillet over medium - high heat and barbecue or sear chicken fillets on each side until golden, crispy and cooked through. Once chicken is cooked, set aside and allow to rest.

Slice chicken into strips and get ready plate of mixed greens with lettuce, avocado slices, tomatoes, mozzarella cheese and chicken. Top with basil strips; drizzle with the remaining dressing; season with salt and pepper; serve.

36. 10 MINUTE PORTOBELLO PIZZAS

These pizzas are fast and easy to make, low carb and ready in 10 minutes! SERVES: 6\sINGREDIENTS

6 portobello mushroom covers, stems removed, washed and dried with a paper towel

2 tablespoons extra virgin olive oil 2 teaspoons minced garlic

6 teaspoons Italian seasoning (or a dried oregano and basil leaf blend), divided

3/4 cup pizza sauce (garlic and herb) (garlic and herb)

1 1/2 cups reduced-fat shredded mozzarella cheese (or a pizza cheese blend)* 30 miniature-sized pepperonis**\s6 cherry or grape tomatoes, cut thinly Salt and pepper, to taste

INSTRUCTIONS

Preheat broiler to broil/grill settings on high heat. Arrange oven shelf to the middle of your oven.

Combine the oil, garlic and 4 teaspoons of the seasoning together in a little bowl. Brush the bottoms of each mushroom with the garlic oil mixture and place each mushroom, oil side down, on a softly greased baking sheet/tray.

Fill each mushroom with 2 tablespoons of the pizza sauce per cap, 1/4 cup of mozzarella cheddar, 6 pepperoni miniatures and tomato cuts. Broil/grill until cheese has softened and is brilliant in colour (about 8 minutes) (about 8 minutes).

To serve, sprinkle with the staying Italian seasoning (or mixed herbs), and season with salt and pepper to taste.

CONCLUSION

Widely shifting degrees of sugar intake have been effective for the target outcomes of improved glycemic control and reduced CVD risk among individuals with diabetes. In any case, hereditary and other factors may impact reaction in people at hazard for or with diabetes.

While protein is a very important dietary component , too much protein can be destructive. Additionally, protein from the wrong source can have major negative wellbeing consequences. Not only does protein from animal based sources contribute to heart disease, however the baggage that it carries with it, namely cholesterol and immersed fat, significantly adds to heart infection development as well.

Aim to get your protein exclusively from plant based sources . There is no such thing as a protein deficiency as long as a variety of whole plant foods is consumed and enough calories are eaten.Gumbo with shrimp and sausage (nineteenth) 30 minute prep 1 hr 30 min to prepare

8 servings (approximately).

509 cals

INGREDIENTS

1 pound raw shrimp, peeled and deveined 4 smoked Andouille sausage links (approximately 12 ounces) 2 red and orange bell peppers, chopped 1 yellow onion, chopped

20 carrots, baby-cut (about 1 cup) 28 oz. squashed tomatoes 5 scallions, sliced 4 cup broth de poulet

To prepare the roux, combine the following ingredients in a blender and blend until smooth.

all-purpose flour, 1/2 cup 1 teaspoon of butter

Canola oil (1/4 cup)

F or a cajun seasoning mixture:

2 tsp garlic powder 1 tsp dried thyme paprika, 2 tblsp.

1 teaspoon dry minced onion 2 teaspoons salt 1 teaspoon cayenne pepper

1 tsp chili powder

INSTRUCTIONS

To make the cajun seasoning, combine all of the following ingredients in a small mixing bowl. In a small mixing bowl, combine and mix the cajun fixings. Remove the item from circulation.

To make the roux, combine all of the ingredients in a mixing bowl and whisk In a large pot or dutch oven (at least 5 quarts), heat the canola oil over medium heat. Combine the flour and the spread. Cook, stirring constantly, for about 15 minutes, or until the roux turns a dull caramel shade.

Add the bell peppers, onions, and carrots to the pot with the roux to cook. Stir in the roux until it's completely mixed in. Cook for 10 minutes, stirring occasionally, until the vegetables have softened and become fragrant.

Add liquids and spices to the pot to simmer: Combine the squashed tomatoes (including liquid), chicken broth, and salt and pepper in a large mixing bowl.

to the equivalent pot, add the scallions and cajun seasoning Bring to a boil, then reduce to a medium heat and allow to simmer. Allow for 1 hour of simmering time after covering with a lid.

Uncover the pot and add shrimp and hotdog. In the same pot, combine the shrimp and wiener. Allow about 5 minutes for the shrimp to become opaque and cooked. Remove the pan from the heat and serve immediately with rice.

Soup with No Tortillas (no tortilla) (no tortillas) (no tortillas) (no tortillas

Remove the seeds from the jalapeos before dicing them if you don't like spicy foods.

INGREDIENTS

1 tbsp. ghee (clarified butter) (explained butter) 1 large, diced yellow onion 6 peeled and minced garlic cloves

2 diced new jalapeos (and cultivated, if you wish) chicken stock (two quarts) Fire-roasted tomatoes, 11 oz.

1 cooked and diced pound of chicken breast a cup of chopped fresh cilantro two limes (juice)

To serve, garnish with avocado slices, lime pinwheels, or fresh cilantro minced.

DIRECTIONS

Ghee should be heated over medium heat in a Dutch stove or soup pot. Cook for 4 to 6 minutes, or until onions are clear.

Garlic and jalapeo peppers should be added at this point. 1–2 minutes, or until fragrant Bring the chicken stock and tomatoes to a medium boil, then reduce to a low heat and cook for 3–5 minutes.

Stir in the cooked chicken, cilantro, and lime juice until everything is well combined. Enjoy the soup with whatever garnish you like!

31. CILANTRO AND LIME CHICKEN AND AVOCADO SALAD

4 SERVINGS YIELDS

15 MINUTES FOR PREPARE 15 MINUTES TOTAL WORK TIME

The flavors in this Low-Carb Chicken and Avocado Salad with Lime and Cilantro are superb.

INGREDIENTS

2 c. cooked chicken, shredded into huge chunks 2 t fresh lime juice 2 medium avocados, diced to taste with salt

1 cup green onion, thinly sliced

fresh cilantro, finely chopped (or chop it more coarsely if you prefer)

INSTRUCTIONS

Shred the chicken into large chunks until you have 2 cups.

Avocados should be diced into medium-sized pieces, then mixed with 1 tablespoon lime juice and salt to taste.

Green onion, thinly sliced, and cilantro, finely chopped To make the dressing, whisk together 1 tablespoon mayonnaise and 1 teaspoon lime juice.

Place the chicken in a large mixing bowl that can accommodate all of the salad ingredients. Toss in the sliced green onions and the dressing until the chicken is thoroughly coated.

In the bottom of the bowl, combine the avocado and any lime juice with the chicken and toss tenderly.

Then, just barely combine the chopped cilantro with the salad.

Serve right away or chill until ready to serve. This could be served in pita bread, sandwich bread, or lettuce cups, but we just ate it as a salad.

I'm sure it'll keep in the fridge for a few days, but I didn't have any when I made it!

32. EGG CUPS WITH CAULIFLOWER HASH 15 MINUTES TO PREPARE AND 20 MINUTES TO COOK

35 MINUTES TOTAL

12 PARTS

INGREDIENTS

1 cauliflower head, cut into florets with the stalk and leaves removed furthermore 1 whisked large egg

cheddar cheese, 1/2 cup (or Mozzarella) Parmesan cheese, grated

Parmesan cheese, grated salt, 1 teaspoon (to your tastes) cayenne (optional -to taste)

garlic powder (1/2 teaspoon) (or 1 teaspoon onion powder) 12 medium-sized eggs, 12 small eggs

INSTRUCTIONS

Preheat the oven to 230°C | 350°F. Lightly spray a 12-hole muffin tin with cooking oil splash (or butter) and set aside.

Pulse the cauliflower in two clumps for 30 – 50 seconds, or until a fine 'rice' forms. If there are a few larger pieces in there, that's fine. (If you process the cauliflower too much, it will turn into a raw puree.)

In a microwave-safe bowl, measure out 3 cups (480g or 17oz) cauliflower rice and heat for about 8 minutes or until soft. Alternatively, lightly steam over a pot of boiling water or in a vegetable steamer until soft. Eliminate and allow to cool for a good 5 minutes before handling.

Using paper towels , an old tea towel or a cheesecloth, squeeze out as much liquid as you can until hardly any liquid can be squeezed out. (It's simpler to wrap the cauliflower in the towel (or cloth) and squeeze it into a ball over the sink. Less mess)

Transfer back into your bowl (make sure there's no liquid in it), and add the whisked egg, cheeses, salt and garlic powder. Divide the blend into each muffin hole and firmly press them with your fingertips to create a 'nest' or cup.

Bake for about 15 -20 minutes or until the cheddar has softened, the cups are brilliant and the edges are browned. Remove from the oven; break the eggs into each cup; season with salt and pepper; return to the oven and bake for an into each cup; season with salt and pepper; return to the oven and bake for a 15 minutes, or until the whites are set and the yolks are cooked to your liking.

Allow them to cool for 5 minutes before handling them , or they may fall apart. Lightly slide a blade around the sides of each cup. Utilizing a fork, delicately lift one side first to make sure they're not sticking to the bottom, and lift out of the pan.

Garnish with red chilli flakes and parsley (discretionary) or leave as is.

33. ORANGE CHICKEN LETTUCE WRAPS

Prep time: 5 MINS Cook time: 15 MINS Total time: 20 MINS

Easy to make, light and healthy orange chicken lettuce wraps! The ground chicken tastes just like a healthier form of orange chicken and being in lettuce wraps means it's a low carb, high protein, filling meal for lunch or dinner.

INGREDIENTS:

ORANGE CHICKEN SAUCE:

1/2 cup orange juice 1tablespoons orange zest 2 tablespoons soy sauce

2tablespoons apple cider vinegar 1/4 cup brown sugar

1 teaspoon garlic, minced

1/2 teaspoon EACH ground ginger AND red pepper flakes 2 tablespoons water AND 1/2 tablespoons cornstarch

CHICKEN FILLING:

1 tablespoon oil

1 pound ground chicken (turkey or beef works too) (turkey or beef works too) 2 teaspoons garlic, minced

1 (10. 5 ounce) can mandarin oranges (new dollface slices work too) (new dollface slices work too) cleaved scallions, lettuce leaves AND toasted sesame seeds for decorating ORANGE CHICKEN SAUCE: Combine the

elements for the sauce in an artisan jar, give it a few good shakes until all the ingredients are blended. Pour the sauce into a small pan and heat over medium high heat. When the sauce begins to stew, lower the heat and allow to cook for an extra 1-2 minutes. You need the sauce to be thick enough to coat the back of a spoon. Remove from stove, allow to cool.

CHICKEN FILLING: Heat the oil in a large skillet over medium-high heat. Add the ground chicken and break down any lumps with a wooden spoon, then add the garlic and let the chicken cook for 5-7 minutes or until it cooks all the way through. Sprinkle the chicken with the prepared sauce. Let cook for 1-2 minutes. Adjust with salt and pepper to taste. Allow the filling to cool for several minutes before filling lettuce leaves. Top with mandarin orange cuts and toasted sesame seeds.

34. GARLIC BUTTER BAKED SALMON IN FOIL Prep time: 5 MINS Cook time: 20 MINS

Total time: 25 MINS

Garlic spread baked salmon in no time at all! Start with a straightforward lemon garlic margarine sauce that's super fancy yet also truly easy to make then we just pour this on top of a filet of salmon and prepare it off in the oven wrapped in foil. The salmon is flakey and delicate this way, and the garlic butter flavor is out of this world!

INGREDIENTS:\s1¼ pound sockeye or coho salmon (ideally wild caught)* 2 tablespoons EACH: lemon juice AND cold butter, cubed 2cloves garlic, minced\s½ teaspoon salt

¼ teaspoon EACH: Italian seasoning, red pepper chips AND black pepper 1 tablespoon hacked parsley, for embellishing (optional) (optional)

PREP: Position a rack in the center of the oven and preheat the oven to 375°F.

SAUCE: In a saucepan over medium heat, combine the lemon juice and minced garlic, permit the lemon juice to reduce to 1 tablespoon. Add in 1 tablespoon of butter, remove pan from heat and swirl so the butter begins to melt. Place back on the hotness for a few seconds, removed and continue to swirl until butter totally melts. Repeat with second tablespoon of butter. When butter is completely liquefied, add the Italian preparing, red pepper flakes, salt and pepper. Then, remove sauce from stove.

BAKE: Place the salmon filet in a piece of foil large enough to overlap over and seal. Utilizing a brush or spoon, brush the salmon with the garlic spread sauce. Cover with foil so that all sides are properly closed so the sauce doesn't leak. Bake the salmon for 12-14 minutes or until mostly firm to the touch.

Open the foil and allow the fish to cook under the oven for 2-3 minutes, keeping an eye on it so the fish doesn't consume. Remove from oven, top with parsley. Serve immediately.

35. CHICKEN AVOCADO CAPRESE SALAD

Balsamic Chicken Avocado Caprese Salad is a fast and simple meal in a plate of mixed greens! Seared chicken, fresh mozzarella and tomato parts, creamy avocado cuts and shredded basil

leaves are sprinkled with an unimaginable balsamic dressing that doubles as a marinade for the ultimate salad!

PREP: 5 MINS

COOK: 15 MINS

TOTAL: 20 MINS

SERVES: 4

INGREDIENTS

Marinade/Dressing:\s1/4 cup (60 mL) (60 mL) balsamic vinegar 2 tablespoons (30 mL) olive oil

2 teaspoons brown sugar 1 teaspoon minced garlic 1 teaspoon dried basil

1 teaspoon salt

S alad:\s4chicken thigh fillets, skin removed (no bone)*\s5cups Romaine, (or cos) lettuce leaves, washed and dried 1 avocado, sliced\s1 cup cherry or grape tomatoes, sliced

1/2 cup mini mozzarella/bocconcini cheddar balls 1/4 cup basil leaves, thinly sliced

Salt and pepper, to season

INSTRUCTIONS

Whisk marinade ingredients together to combine . Place chicken into a shallow dish; pour 4 tablespoons of the dressing/marinade onto the chicken and stir around to equally coat chicken. Reserve the untouched marinade to use as a dressing.

Heat about one teaspoon of oil in a large grill dish or skillet over medium - high heat and barbecue or sear chicken fillets on each side until golden, crispy and cooked through. Once chicken is cooked, set aside and allow to rest.

Slice chicken into strips and get ready plate of mixed greens with lettuce, avocado slices, tomatoes, mozzarella cheese and chicken. Top with basil strips; drizzle with the remaining dressing; season with salt and pepper; serve.

36. 10 MINUTE PORTOBELLO PIZZAS

These pizzas are fast and easy to make, low carb and ready in 10 minutes! SERVES: 6\sINGREDIENTS

6 portobello mushroom covers, stems removed, washed and dried with a paper towel

2 tablespoons extra virgin olive oil 2 teaspoons minced garlic

6 teaspoons Italian seasoning (or a dried oregano and basil leaf blend), divided

3/4 cup pizza sauce (garlic and herb) (garlic and herb)

1 1/2 cups reduced-fat shredded mozzarella cheese (or a pizza cheese blend)* 30 miniature-sized pepperonis**\s6 cherry or grape tomatoes, cut thinly Salt and pepper, to taste

INSTRUCTIONS

Preheat broiler to broil/grill settings on high heat. Arrange oven shelf to the middle of your oven.

Combine the oil, garlic and 4 teaspoons of the seasoning together in a little bowl. Brush the bottoms of each mushroom with the garlic oil mixture and place each mushroom, oil side down, on a softly greased baking sheet/tray.

Fill each mushroom with 2 tablespoons of the pizza sauce per cap, 1/4 cup of mozzarella cheddar, 6 pepperoni miniatures and tomato cuts. Broil/grill until cheese has softened and is brilliant in colour (about 8 minutes) (about 8 minutes).

To serve, sprinkle with the staying Italian seasoning (or mixed herbs), and season with salt and pepper to taste.

CONCLUSION

Widely shifting degrees of sugar intake have been effective for the target outcomes of improved glycemic control and reduced CVD risk among individuals with diabetes. In any case, hereditary and other factors may impact reaction in people at hazard for or with diabetes.

While protein is a very important dietary component , too much protein can be destructive. Additionally, protein from the wrong source can have major negative wellbeing consequences. Not only does protein from animal based sources contribute to heart disease, however the baggage that it carries with it, namely cholesterol and immersed fat, significantly adds to heart infection development as well.

Aim to get your protein exclusively from plant based sources . There is no such thing as a protein deficiency as long as a variety of whole plant foods is consumed and enough calories are eaten.

Chapter Two

HIGH PROTEIN, LOW CARB FOODS

High -protein, low carb foods can be delectable, too. Atkins has compiled a list of the best sources of protein among low carb snacks and food sources. Peruse on for recipes and products that incorporate these tasty ingredients.

1. Fish

Certain types of seafood are lauded as protein powerhouses , such as yellowfin tuna, halibut, and tilapia. Try Bahian Halibut, a well-seasoned Caribbean dish with coconut flavors; it offers 48.7g of protein, 18.6g of fat, 1.1g of fiber, 4.6g of net carbs, and 400 calories per serving. Bring Tuna-Celery Salad to lunch and enjoy a protein-filled noontime feast; one serving offers 37g of protein.

2. Tofu

Tofu is an excellent vegetarian protein to add to a dish as it easily absorbs whatever flavors it's cooked with. Flavor up heated tofu with a zesty kick such as a chipotle marinade or a Moroccan rub. For a savory Meatless Monday supper, try Tofu Pad Thai, which contains 20.5g of protein, 26.9g of fat, 6.9g of fiber, 14.1g of net carbs, and 374.6 calories.

3. Eggs

The poster child of protein , one egg offers 6g of complete protein. This means it gives all the amino acids humans need in their diet. Jump start your day with a protein-packed dish such as Eggs Scrambled with Cheddar, Swiss Chard and Canadian Bacon. This entrée includes 32.6g of protein, 36.9g of fat, 1.2g of fiber, 3.6g of net carbs, and 482.9 calories.

4. Nuts

Nuts are a high protein , low carb snack that offer heart-solid fats and a lot of protein. In particular, peanuts, cashews, and almonds are great wagers for high-protein snacks. The Atkins Chocolate Peanut Butter Pretzel Bar packs a whopping 16g of protein between nibbles of real roasted peanuts, pretzels, and smooth peanut butter. You can also snatch a small bunch of Atkins Sweet and Salty Trail Mix, which is equal parts salty and sweet, with 7g of protein.

5. Chicken

Chicken is a great high protei n food. For dinner, try Green Goddess Grilled Chicken, which packs in 53g of protein, 16.9g of fat, 1.4g of net carbs, and 382.4calories Chicken Salad makes for a filling lunch, thanks to over 50g of protein per serving. Use a lettuce wrap for an added crunch.

Chapter Three

WHAT YOU CAN AND CAN'T EAT

For protein, you can eat fish, poultry, red meat, low-fat cheddar (cottage cheese, feta, mozzarella, Muenster), eggs, and tofu.

Also permitted: leafy green vegetables, tomatoes, peppers, broccoli, eggplant, zucchini, green beans, asparagus, celery, cucumber, and mushrooms.

The plan calls for you to get 25 grams of fiber every day . (For comparison, one cup of whole wheat spaghetti has 6 grams of fiber.) You can likewise have some fats: olive and nut oils, avocado, and butter.

You can have diet sodas and counterfeit sweeteners in moderation. A glass of wine or a light brew is OK, yet their carbs count, too.

To round out nutritional needs, the authors recommend taking a high -quality vitamin- andmineral supplement, along with at least 90 milligrams of potassium.

Level of Effort: Medium

Like many high-protein, low-carb eats less, you may truly need to change what you're eating while you're on this plan.

Limitations: Low -carb diets cut out a lot of food varieties Packaged foods or meals: None are required.

Inperson meetings: No.

Exercise: Yes, I suggest resistance training, such as weight lifting, to help consume stored fat.

Does It Allow for Dietary Restrictions or Preferences?

Vegetarians and vegetarians: This diet could work for you, however you would be eating a lot of tofu for the protein.

Wh at Else You Should Know Cost: No costs apart from the food you buy.

Support: The Protein Power site includes a gathering, in case you need to get in touch with other people on this diet.

A high -protein diet will help you lose weight. A number of studies show that slims down higher in protein keep you fuller better than different sorts of eats less carbs. Other concentrates on show that confining carbs, as a result of a high-protein diet, causes more weight loss. But calories still count!

Is It Good for Certain Conditions?

The Protein Power diet would work for people with diabetes , high blood pressure, heart disease,

or elevated cholesterol. The Power Protein diet is a low-carb diet with less than 20 percent of total calories from carbs or less than 100 grams of carbs each day. Limiting carbs assists lower with blooding sugar, insulin, bad cholesterol, and blood pressure. It likewise boosts HDL ("good") cholesterol.

But getting too much protein can raise your uric acid levels, which can cause gout. Too much protein load also could be a problem in anybody with kidney problems.

You also need to make sure that you're not getting too much fat from your food if your doctor has given you guidelines on that to help lower your cholesterol, for instance.

Women of childbearing age need folate, which is added to flour, and if you cut out carbs, that will mean you get less folate. Prepregnancy weight loss is best finished with a more adjusted methodology that cuts calories.

It 's a simple dieting approach that basically disposes of one major food group, and, as any restrictive diet, it is difficult for most people to sustain for a long time.

This eating routine will help you lose weight, however if you have a particular nutritional need this may not be the diet for you. You may need to take a daily supplement to cover any nutritional gaps in vitamins and minerals.

Chapter Four

RISKS OF HIGH PROTEIN, LOW CARB DIETS

High protein, low carb diets do have risks these range from normal side effects to more serious long-term health impacts.

Some of the common side impacts reported by people on high protein, low carb diets are:

Bad breath: When there is not enough sugar in your diet, the body needs to transform proteins and fats into carbohydrates. In the process acetone vapours are released making your breath (and wind) smelly.

Constipation: Having too much protein and not enough fiber (from wholegrains, legumes, natural products and vegetables), can make you feel uncomfortable and constipated.

Lack of energy and peevishness: Wholegrain carbs help to fuel your body and keep your energy levels at their best.

Cutting your carbs will depart you feeling tired, restless and less spurred to do your afternoon rec center session.

Serious health impacts

Along with these more commonly reported side effects, there are more serious health concerns with high protein, low carb consumes less calories. These include:

Your bones . Too much protein can increase calcium loss in your urine, and it may increase your danger of osteoporosis, especially if you don't have enough calcium in your diet.

Your heart. Too much immersed fat from the fat on meat, full-cream dairy products, coconut fat, spread and ghee can clog blood vessels and increase your hazard of heart disease. A review showed that following a high protein, low carb paleo diet for over 10 weeks can increase your awful 'LDL' cholesterol by 20 per cent and decrease your good 'HDL' cholesterol even when exercising!

Your kidneys . A high protein consumption makes your kidneys work harder, which will contribute to the decline in kidney work if you have kidney problems.

Your mind. A high intake of red meat and full-cream dairy products and a reduction of wholegrains, legumes, fruits and vegetables can increase your brain's risk of diseases like Alzheimer's and dementia.

Your life expectancy . According to a new study, reducing your protein intake may also increase your life expectancy and slow down aging.

Cancer hazard. Counts calories high in red meat and low in defensive plant foods are linked with an increased hazard of disease, especially colon cancer.

Diabetes risk. Late research also recommends that slims down high in red meat may also increment your risk of type 2 diabetes.

Because of these risks there are a few gatherings of people who should definitely avoid high protein diets. This includes people who are inclined to kidney stones, have kidney disease or impaired kidney function; people with gout, diabetes, high blood cholesterol or high blood pressure; and people who are pregnant or breastfeeding. However, it's best you speak to your doctor if you're unsure.

So while high protein, low carb diets can work for weight reduction in the present moment, it is definitely not worth harming your health for in the long-term. There is an alternative!

Chapter Five

A WHOLICIOUS APPROACH TO HEALTHY EATING

Don 't be afraid of carbs! Just pick the right ones. The kind of sugars in your diet matter, as do your segment sizes. In the event that you need to lose weight, adhere to the recommended serving sizes and number of serves per day. Also pick wholegrain or wholemeal breads, high fibre cereals and brown rice, in spot of refined sugars from foods such as white bread, highly handled grains and white rice. Vegetarians who based their meals on good quality carbs are the healthiest groups of people in the world.

Choose plant proteins . On the off chance that you want to increase the sum of protein you eat, attempt doing it with more plant proteins, like vegetables and pulses. Not only will they help fill you up, they are one of the foods most associated with living a longer, better life.

Healthy fats . Just like with proteins and carbs, including more sound fats in your eating routine, as those in avocados, nuts and olive oil, can be a decent way to fill you up, help oversee your weight and reduce your coronary illness risk.

Get active . Moving more is an important way of keeping a healthy weight. Fruitful weight misfortune is best accomplished by aiming for an hour most days in your week. In the event that that sounds daunting, start with 20- minute sessions and progressively develop your exercise time as you get fitter.

THE PROTEIN POWER DIET

The diet is fundamentally a low -carb, high-protein eating plan with a ton of scientific explanations about insulin and glucagons, the major hormones that turn food into fuel for your body.

The idea is that by restricting carbs, you lower your insulin level . That leads your body to make more glucagon, which helps consume stored fat. Do this long enough, and the fat seems to melt away.

CPSIA information can be obtained
at www.ICGtesting.com
Printed in the USA
BVHW012348130322
631391BV00008B/401